Abdominal Strength for Life® *!*

A Leaner and Stronger Core After 40, After 65, & Beyond…

Dr. Josef Arnould,

Author of

American Diet Revolution!

***Neck Strength for Life*®**
and
Stronger After 40

Director of

Strength for Life® Health and Fitness Center

Easthampton, Massachusetts

StrengthForLife.com

Abdominal Strength for Life®!

A Leaner and Stronger Core After 40, After 65, and Beyond…

© 2018 Josef Arnould, D.C.

Published in Easthampton, Massachusetts by Strength for Life® Health & Fitness Center. Strength for Life® is a registered U.S. Trademark of CX Associates of Northampton, Inc. www.StrengthForLife.com

ISBN 978-1-7921570-7-3 Paperback

ISBN 978-0-9989617-3-6 eBook

Cover Design by Alan Robinson

Interior Photographs by Alan Robinson and Sarah Whiteley

Interior Illustrations by Josef Arnould, DC, Ella Boliver, and Alan Robinson

Editing and Proofreading by Ellen Marie Deehan-Magnone

Digital Layout and Design by Sami Shields of Smart to Finish Divas

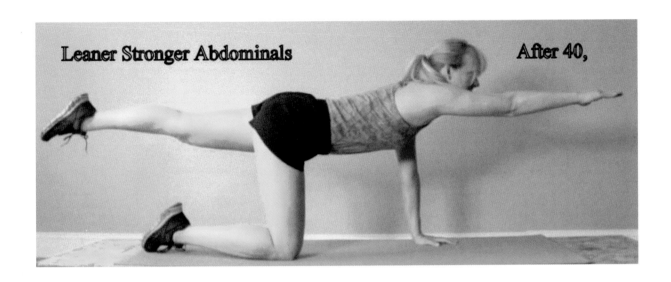

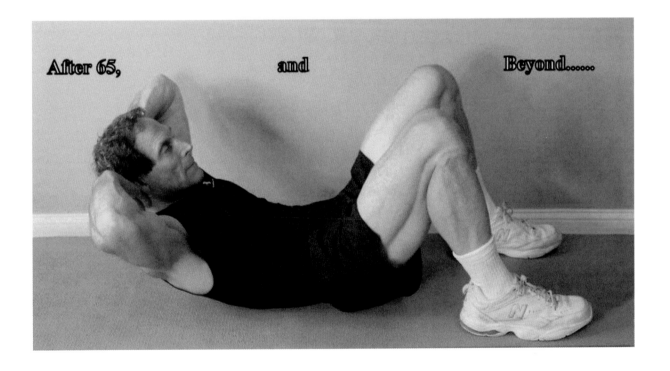

This is a work dedicated to

Anyone and Everyone

Desiring to Be

Leaner,

Stronger,

and Healthier

Throughout Adulthood.

Table of Contents

Introduction   7

Part I: *The Foundation for Phenomenal Abdominals*

    Chapter 1: What Are the Core Muscles?   14
    Chapter 2: Why Not Strength for Life®?   24
    Chapter 3: Meet Your Abdominals
           and Their Sidekicks   28

Part II: *The Abdominal Strength for Life® Program*

    Chapter 4: Beginning Level
           Abdominal Medley #1   54
    Chapter 5: Intermediate Level
           Abdominal Medley #2   75
    Chapter 6: Intermediate Level
           Abdominal Medley #3   91

Part III: *Leaner for Life*

    Chapter 7: The American Diet Revolution   109
    Chapter 8: Cardiorespiratory Conditioning   117
    Chapter 9: Whole-Body Strength for Life®
           Training   122
Coda   136

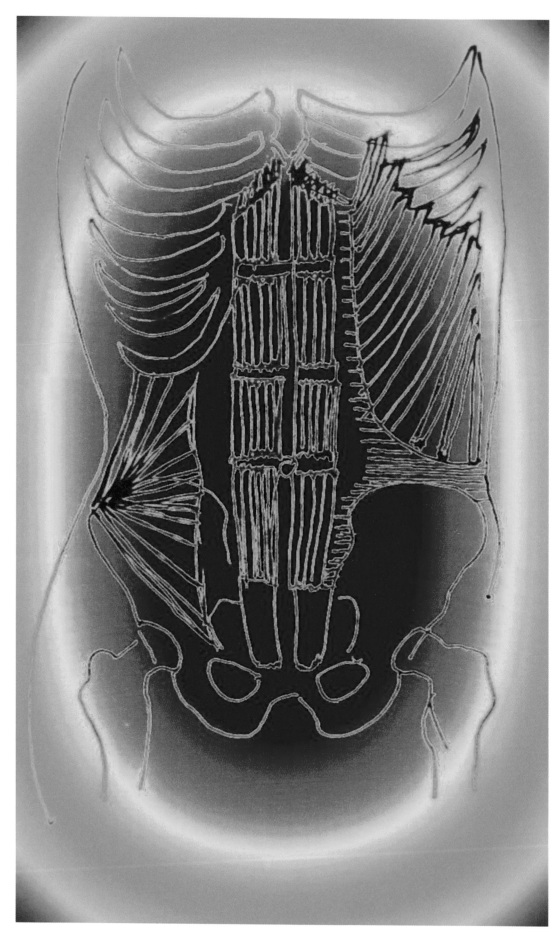

Introduction

You, as most of us who are American adults, want to develop and maintain a trim and strong midsection of your body. Several important motivating factors drive you to accomplish this goal.

First, a trim waist bolsters your self-image—how you see yourself—both in your mind, when your eyes are closed, and in the mirror, when they are open. When you see and feel yourself as lean and strong, your self-confidence rises. Every day, you feel energized and capable of accomplishing the most important goals in your life.

Second, in addition to how you appear to yourself, you care about how you appear to others. How other people view you affects your chances to be hired for a job, to be approved for a bank loan, to be attractive to a potential partner, even to receive courteous counter service at a store.

Third, in the back of your mind, you know that having a lean midsection of your body is one sign of good health. We have all heard ominous health statistics: more than 2/3 of American adults are obese or seriously overweight; being obese compounds your risk to become diabetic; being diabetic doubles your risk to develop dementia. Having a lean waist does not guarantee you will not be afflicted with any of these disorders; however, it reduces greatly the probability that you will be.

A fourth—and perhaps the most important—motivation to develop a lean and strong midsection is that it feels great! Your clothes fit comfortably. You feel capable of excelling in your favorite physical activities. You are not afraid you are going to injure your back whenever you are physically active. When you walk or run, you feel the core muscles of your lower torso gyrating gracefully around your waist and hips. When you rotate your body to hit a golf ball or rake leaves, you feel power in your abdominal and hip muscles. You feel fabulous!

Ironically, despite a strong desire to develop leaner and stronger abdominals—and many good reasons to do so—most of us do not succeed in this quest. Why are we failing?

Over the past 35 years, I have taught "core" muscle exercises to thousands of patients and wellness exercise clients in the Strength for Life® Health & Fitness Center. Based upon this experience, I believe there are several gaps in crucial information which are preventing most of us—maybe including you—from accomplishing the goal of having a leaner and stronger midsection. Four of the most important of these informational gaps are:

1. Although most of us have a picture in mind about what good "abs" look like, many of us do not have a clear definition of what the "core" muscles are and where they are located. "Are the "core" muscles just the abdominal muscles? What are the "muffin tops"? Are they muscles too? Or are they just a place where fat accumulates?"

2. Many of us are also uncertain about the functions of "core" muscles. "What do these muscles actually do? Do they just hold my waist in? Does getting them stronger always mean my waistline will be smaller?

3. Most Americans are extremely confused about <u>the types of foods we should avoid—to decrease excess fat in our bodies—as well as the types of foods we should add to our diets—if we want to develop a lean and muscular waistline</u>. In addition, a surprisingly large number of people believe, "If I can just do a lot of cardio exercise, that will lower my body fat and I won't have to worry much about what I am eating."

4. Very few of us have discovered and stayed consistent with a well-organized, systematic, "core" muscle development program that takes us from the simplest—but most essential—abdominal strengthening exercises right up to the most challenging ones for all the "core" muscle groups. Instead, we see a 22-year-old bodybuilder on a TV infomercial, and say to ourselves, "Now that is what I want!" In taking this bait, however, we are only looking at a finished product. We have very little insight into the essential steps one must master in order to reach such an advanced degree of fitness. Purchasing the latest exercise gizmo demonstrated by a model on a television screen will not guide you through the fundamentals of core training you must take to achieve your personal goals for strength and leanness. The book you are now reading will!

The primary purpose of *Abdominal Strength for Life®!* is to present you with a well-organized system of "core" muscle strengthening exercises and to help you overcome information gaps 1 to 4. The present book is the first of a two-volume set. In this volume, you are guided through the Beginning and Intermediate Levels of the Abdominal Strength for Life® program. I have developed this step-by-step plan from experience gained while teaching thousands of people of all ages and all levels of physical fitness. When you work your way up gradually through a sequence of exercises of increasing difficulty, you will achieve your goals for abdominal strength and middle-of-the-body leanness. However, before you start to perform these exercises, it is essential that you begin to fill in information gaps 1 and 2. To truly master intricate core exercises, you must define as precisely as possible the words you are using and the goals you are pursuing.

Part I of this volume, which includes the first three chapters, is entitled, "The Foundation for Phenomenal Abdominals." In Chapter 1, *"What Are the Core Muscles,"* we define and differentiate the terms "abdominal muscles" and "core muscles." These are related, but not synonymous. Next, we must define three other key words used in the title and subtitle of this book.

What does "leaner" mean?
What is "strength"?
How do you know if your core muscles are "stronger"?

In Chapter 2, "Why Not Strength for Life?", we address another important health concern for almost all of us: gaining extra body fat as we age. Between 25 and 55, the average American adult accumulates 45 additional pounds of body fat and loses approximately 15 pounds of muscle and bone. "For Life" is the key.

So why does the subtitle say, "After 40?"
Why "After 65?"
"And Beyond?" (Are you kidding me?)

In Chapter 3, "Meet the Abdominals and Their Sidekicks," you'll take a brief anatomical tour of the "core" muscles and their actions. To succeed in your exercise efforts, you must have at least a rudimentary picture in your mind of the muscles you are challenging and the movements they can create. This chapter concludes with "The Fundamentals of Core Exercise Execution," a clear list of the vital exercise techniques you can use to improve the efficiency of every core exercise you perform.

Practicing these principles enables you to squeeze as much benefit and joy as possible out of every moment you invest in your personal training programs.

Part II of this volume, comprising the middle three chapters, is entitled "The Abdominal Strength for Life® Program: Beginning and Intermediate Levels." With detailed instructions and precise photographs, you will be guided through three separate "core" muscle workouts.

In Chapter 4, "Abdominal Medley #1," you will learn, practice, and perfect six fundamental exercises. Some of these exercises may seem simple at first. Soon, however, you will discover there is an enormous difference between merely rattling off numerous repetitions of an exercise versus focusing intently upon your target muscles as you savor every millimeter of movement in every repetition of that exercise. You will perceive this great difference because in the first three chapters you will have begun to fill in informational gaps 1 and 2. You will have a picture in your mind of the precise muscle groups you are exercising and how these muscles function.

As you master the exercises in Chapter 4, you will be amazed at how quickly you feel changes in your body. You will wake up with fewer aches and pains. Your pants will feel a little looser around the belt line. You will feel stronger and more flexible when you carry packages, climb a ladder, or swing a golf club. Some people are so satisfied with the results they achieve just by performing these fundamental exercises, that they are content to continue training only at this beginning level.

You, on the other hand—as well as many of the rest of us—may be aiming for an even higher degree of "core" fitness. You are well prepared for this quest. In mastering the beginning level exercises, you established a functional foundation upon which all subsequent and more challenging exercises are based. Virtually all intermediate and advanced core exercises are merely more complicated and more demanding versions of the basic six. This illustrates why learning to perform these beginning exercises with focus and precision is crucial. Even if you believe you are already at an advanced level of abdominal fitness, you can benefit significantly by practicing and perfecting the six beginning exercises in this program before moving on to intermediate and advanced levels of training. Personally, I enjoy performing these beginning exercises with as much precision and concentration as I do the most challenging advanced ones. In my experience, continuing to execute beginning exercises regularly and with concentration, increases my ability to perform intermediate and advanced ones with grace, power, and efficiency.

The Intermediate Level of the Abdominal Strength for Life® Program consists of two separate workouts, which are presented in Chapters 5 and 6, respectively.

In Chapter 5, you will again execute all six of the beginning exercises, but while balancing on an agility ball (AKA: exercise ball, yoga ball, physioball, etc.). Being perched on an agility ball not only creates the opportunity to build great strength, it demands and cultivates enhanced flexibility, coordination, equilibrium, balance and, of course, agility.

In Chapter 6, you are challenged by a second intermediate level core muscle workout. Here you meet a set of floor exercises that are—both physically and mentally—more demanding versions of the six floor exercises you mastered in the Beginning Level workout. Once you have mastered these new exercises, along with those in Chapter 5, you will have attained a very high level of core muscle strength and fitness.

Before previewing the third and final section of this book, I feel compelled to explain why the Advanced Level exercises of the Abdominal Strength for Life® Program are not included in one single comprehensive volume. My answer is simple. The book would be too long! If I inserted all the advanced level abdominal exercises into the present book, it would be more than 200 pages in length. We live in a hectic world. Our attention spans have declined precipitously, even in the past few decades. We favor information delivered in small to moderate doses, rather than in huge packages. A second reason for offering Advanced Level core exercises in a separate volume is that most readers of the present book will accomplish their health and fitness goals simply by mastering the Beginning and Intermediate Levels. The advanced exercises in the Abdominal Strength for Life® Program are very demanding. Only a limited number of people will want to add them to their training plans. However, if you are interested, Volume Two of *Abdominal Strength for Life!* is scheduled for release early in 2019.

After that brief digression, let's return to the present book, Volume One. Part III is entitled "Leaner for Life." It consists of three brief chapters designed to eliminate some of the confusion created by information gap #3. I say some of the confusion, because the topic of each of these chapters is worthy of an entire book. Chapter 7, "The American Diet Revolution," is a summary of 21st Century principles of nutritious eating for strength, leanness, and health. The fields of dietary advice and nutritional research are complicated and explosive, so complicated and so explosive I have just completed an entire book on this subject. *American Diet Revolution!* is being published by Morgan James and will be available in print on February 12, 2019. In present book, as a prelude to the release of *American Diet Revolution*!, Chapter 7 is a concise guide to the foods you should eat—and to the foods you should not eat—in order to attain better health, more strength, and a leaner waistline.

Chapter 8, "Cardiorespiratory Conditioning," and Chapter 9, "Whole-Body Strength for Life® Training", are also only brief guides to complex health disciplines. Like Chapter 7, they are included as summaries of sound health principles and to stimulate you to study these subjects in more depth.

No matter what your age, may this first volume of *Abdominal Strength for Life!* provide you with the information and inspiration you need to attain and maintain leaner and stronger abdominals throughout your entire life!

Josef Arnould, D.C.
Easthampton, Massachusetts
November 2018

Disclaimer

An essential principle set forth in this book is that, prior to making any changes in his or her exercise or dietary habits, each reader is personally responsible to communicate directly and in person with at least one healthcare professional who is knowledgeable in the fields of exercise and nutritional science. The present work advances general guidelines for exercising and eating healthfully. It does not present an exercise prescription for any one specific person. The author assumes no responsibility or liability for such personal use. All persons who read and plan to use the information presented in this book are advised to also discuss their exercise and dietary habits with their personal physician(s).

Part I

The Foundation for Phenomenal Abdominals

Chapter 1   What Are the Core Muscles?

Chapter 2   Why Not Strength for Life®?

Chapter 3   Meet the Abdominals and Their Sidekicks

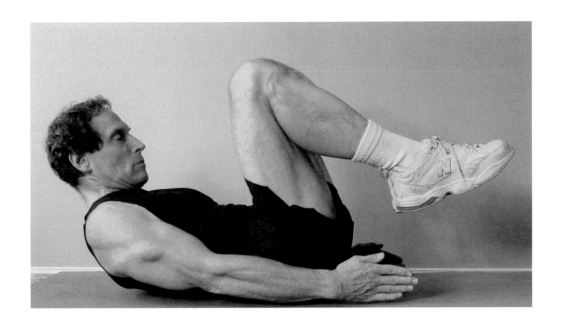

Chapter 1

What Are the Core Muscles?

At some point in adult life, most of us say to ourselves, "I have to strengthen my core." In this moment of personal insight, what precisely do we mean when we use the word "core"?

To many of us, "core" means one specifically located muscle group: the abdominals. We picture clearly defined muscles rippling like corrugated steel and lying sideways across the center of the lower torso. We say to ourselves, "If I could just get my abs to look like that, I would be all set. My core would be super strong. My back would not hurt. I could rake leaves and play golf without any pain. My digestion would be great. I wouldn't have to worry about my weight at all. My clothes would look great on me. My blood pressure would be right on the money…"

Others of us have a more three-dimensional mental picture of the "core." Those of us in this group believe the "core" includes the muscles on the sides of the lower torso—sometimes hidden beneath "muffin tops" or "love handles"—and the muscles of the lower back. We see the "core" as wrapping around the entire circumference of the midsection, like the fibrous and seedy core of an apple after we have eaten the fleshy fruit surrounding it.

Clearly, this second definition of our core muscles is more comprehensive than one limited to only the abdominals. However, even this second mental snapshot of our core may be too restricted. There may be more to the core than we see, at least at first glance.

In addition to assessing the physical appearance and anatomical locations of skeletal muscles, it is vital that we consider also how our muscles function. In thinking about the functions of the muscles of our arms, for instance, we need to consider not just the movements of the biceps and triceps, but also how these two muscle groups interact with movements in the forearm muscles below and in the shoulder muscles above. Hundreds of the physical acts we perform every day require intricate interactions among all these highly related muscle groups. Similarly, in the midsection of the human body, many of the muscular movements of the abdominals and lower back require synchronous movements in the muscles of the hips. For example, the seemingly simple but deceptively complex act of walking requires highly coordinated movements among all the major muscle groups above <u>and</u> below the waist.

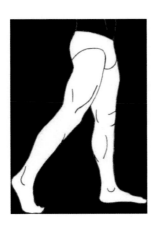 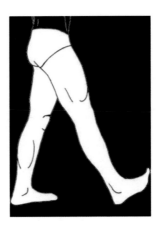

A truly functional definition of our "core" must include all the muscles around the entire circumference of the human body from the bottom of the rib cage to the tops of the knees. Thus, another term we may use to describe our "core" is the Lower Torso/Hip Complex. The muscles that create movements in the hip joints work in intricate harmony with those that create movements in the lower torso. In this comprehensive view of our "core," we see a motion picture. We visualize highly coordinated actions in all the major muscles in the middle third of our bodies as we engage in thousands of physical activities every day of our lives.

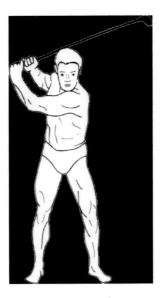

Once you have established in your mind's eye a comprehensive and functional understanding of the core muscles, you can create dozens of new exercises, enabling you to perform a myriad of graceful and powerful movements they make possible.

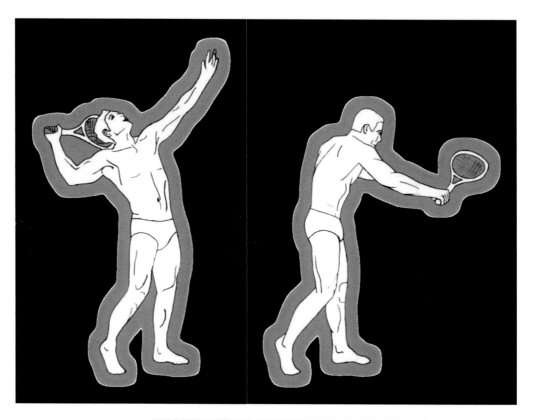

Looking ahead, in Chapter 3 you will review illustrations and the movements of all the essential muscle groups in the Lower Torso/Hip complex. As you progress through

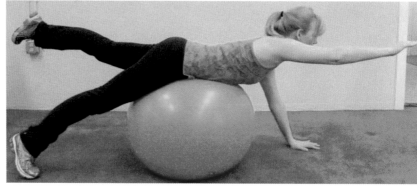

Chapters 4, 5, and 6, you will enjoy many exercises that challenge all your highly interrelated core muscles. Now that is exercise excitement!

What Does "Leaner" Mean?

The comparative adjective "Leaner," as used in the subtitle of this book, is a declaration that: (1) striving for a healthy level of body fat is an important personal goal for each of us; and (2), by eating and exercising intelligently, you can progress toward this goal throughout your entire lifetime.

Many people use a bathroom scale to measure their progress in the struggle to become and remain lean as they age. However, **"leaner" means much more than simply reducing one's gross body weight. "Leaner" denotes each person's individual potential to lower his or her percent body fat** today, tomorrow, and as far into the future as possible. This distinction is crucial. Even if your body weight has remained the same since high school, it is highly probable that the percentage of you which is fat has increased significantly. We human beings never stay the same, not for one day. Each day we age, we become fatter or leaner, stronger or weaker, stiffer or more flexible.

Becoming leaner is a quality of health for which we all must strive every day throughout life. If your body fat percentage is too high now, or even just right, you must exercise and eat well today, if you want to be slightly leaner, as opposed to slightly fatter, tomorrow. By eating and exercising intelligently every day, you will become a little leaner in a month and much leaner in a year. Considering "leaner" from this point of view, several important points obtain.

1. **Do not** compare yourself or your current percent body fat to anyone else, only to yourself.
2. **Do not** compare yourself to who you were 20, 30, or 40 years ago.
3. **Do** compare yourself today to the person you will become in 3, 6, 9, or 12 months. If you have extra fat around your waistline now, you can definitely be visibly leaner and have a smaller waistline circumference in six months to twelve months. Qualitative measurements will confirm this.

4. **Do** compare yourself to the fatter person you will become in one year if you do not exercise intelligently and eat well. You will always be leaner and healthier than the slacker version of you who does not strive consistently to be leaner, stronger, and in better health.

We humans come in many different sizes and shapes and from many different genetic and environmental backgrounds. Many of us, possibly you, may never described as being "lean." But, by gosh, if you try to eat well, to exercise vigorously, and to follow other healthy habits consistently, you will definitely be much leaner than the person you would have become, if you had not applied yourself so diligently. How intensively you choose to push yourself to become leaner is purely an individual decision. For many of us, just getting down to a respectable belt size and reaching a healthy body fat percentage are all we and our health care providers desire. Mastering just the first one or two levels of core muscle training described in this book—and, of course, eating for well-being—will help you reach this degree of middle-of-the-body fitness.

Before we leave the discussion of becoming "lean" and/or "leaner", we must acknowledge that our diets are pre-eminent in determining if we achieve these goals. In **Why We Get Fat**, distinguished science writer Gary Taubes documents and explains how the qualities of the foods we eat affect the production and release of hormones in our bodies. The effects of these hormones are the most important factors in determining if we gain or lose body fat. Exercising for hours every day will not compensate for a habit of continually eating foods that raise our blood sugar levels quickly and repeatedly. Doing 1000 repetitions of abdominal exercises will not do it. Doing two hours of "cardio" exercises will not do it.

Why?

Routinely eating foods that raise your blood glucose levels rapidly and for extended periods of time prevents the release of hormones that allow you to burn the energy stored in your body fat. Without these hormonal signals, your body will hoard the energy stored in fat cells. Therefore, you must disabuse yourself of the misconception that you can achieve a healthful level of body fat through exercise alone. A great core training program will help you develop incredibly strong and flexible muscles in the midsection of your body. Performing cardiorespiratory and whole-body strength exercises will do the same for all the other important muscles of your body. But to achieve a leaner waistline, you must learn to avoid eating foods that prevent the release of energy stored in your fat cells. Chapter 7 will guide you to the foods you must eat and the foods you must not eat, if you want to shrink your fat cells and become the leaner you.

Measuring Your Abdominal Leanness

How do we determine if we are lean and if, through training, we are becoming leaner? Three simple measurements help us to determine our progress. First, your training advisor or training partner measures around your lower torso at the level of the navel to determine the circumference of your waist. This is a direct measurement of abdominal girth. Second, he or she records your total body weight. This, however, is merely a quantitative measurement; it does not tell you if you are gaining or losing stored body fat. Third, therefore, we use a qualitative measure, the Bioimpedance method*, to obtain a quick and reasonably accurate estimate of your whole-body composition: what percentage of you is adipose—fat tissue—and what percentage is lean body mass—muscle, bone, organs, etc. By recording these three measurements before you begin the *Abdominal Strength for Life*® program and every three or four months thereafter, you can monitor your progress as you strive to attain and retain a healthful degree of whole-body and abdominal leanness. The following is a reprint of an actual progress chart of a 54-year-old male.

Date >	1/24	4/23	7/22	10/29
Waist	39 in	38.5 in	36.5 in	35 in
Body Weight	222 lbs.	218 lbs.	209 lbs.	201 lbs.
% Body Fat	24.9	23.5	21.0	19.6

*A computerized electrical impulse unit manufactured by Chattanooga Co. The skin caliper method is less accurate and more cumbersome.

What is a healthy body fat percentage?

The Body Mass Index (BMI) is a calculation used commonly to determine if a person is at a healthy body weight and, by extension, if he or she has a healthy level of body fat. The BMI, however, is based only upon measures of a person's height and weight. This method does not distinguish between lean body mass—primarily bone and muscle—and fat tissue. I personally have performed qualitative Bioimpedance body fat percentage measurements on two males of the same age, both six feet tall and each weighing 200 pounds. In other words, these two individuals had an identical BMI. In bioimpedance testing, however, male A had just under 10% body fat, indicating he was very lean, while male B was more than 30% body fat, which indicated pathological obesity. Two men with the same BMI, one lean and muscular, the other weak and flabby. So much for the reliability of the BMI.

If the BMI is unreliable, is there a universally accepted standard for a healthful percent body fat? Not exactly. Eminent exercise physiologists and other health experts have proposed standards, but their proposals vary somewhat. Therefore, in my own clinic I have tried to average the proposals of the experts and then combine them with my own observations and measurements of thousands of individuals over the past 30+ years. The table below represents my estimation of a person's health status based upon measurements of his or her percent body fat.

Health Status Relative to % Body Fat Measured by Bioimpedance Testing

Status	Obese	Overweight	Healthy	Lean	Very Lean
Female	>35%	25%-35%	20%-25%	15%-20%	Less than 15%
Male	>30%	20%-30%	15%-20%	10%-15%	Less than 10%

Please regard these figures as approximations for a general population of adults and not as absolute standards to be applied to you or any other specific individual. Each one of us has unique physiological characteristics that may affect how much fat is stored in our cells. However, when used as a general guideline, this table can be a very helpful method to determine if you are making progress. If you are a female and your beginning level of body fat is measured to be 39%, you can be very certain that you are obese. After six months of eating and exercising intelligently, your body fat may measure as 32%. You know right away that you are significantly leaner, that you are still overweight but no longer obese, and that you are headed toward much better health. It is very likely that this drop in your body fat percentage will correlate highly with decreases in your body weight and in the circumference of your waist. You now have objective measurements to confirm you are developing a leaner core. But what about stronger?

What is Strength?

In addition to leaner core muscles, which make your waistline look great, you want stronger core muscles, which make you feel and look even better. But how can you determine if your core muscles are becoming stronger? This task is not as straightforward as making periodic measurements of your weight, waist circumference, or body fat percentage.

"Stronger" is a comparative adjective describing a superior or increasing degree of "strength," a noun which means different things in different circumstances. To athletes, "strength" may denote the ability to push, pull, or lift very heavy weights or to overpower a competitor. When we are viewer/victims of television commercials, we hear the word "strength" used to describe the superlative quality of a certain brand of plastic garbage bag that resists rupture, even when it is fully loaded. To historians, "strength" describes the character of leaders, such as Churchill and FDR, during times of extreme crisis.

Clearly, to determine if your core muscles are becoming stronger, you need a definition of "strength" that you can apply specifically to the integrity and function of your core. The following is a working definition:

> "Strength" of the core muscles is the ability to flex forward and extend backward, and to laterally flex and rotate to each side, the lower torso and hips in powerful and coordinated movements through ranges of motion that are as full as possible.

This is a narrow and mechanical definition of "strength," but also one which is functional and applicable to your immediate needs. The highly variable combination of the specific muscular movements described above determines the strength of your core. As you master many different exercises in the Abdominal Strength for Life® program, you will develop an ever-greater awareness of these muscles and the movements they create.

How Do You Know if Your Core is Becoming Stronger?

In many muscle groups of the human body, we can measure increases in strength by the amount of weight we can lift. This is the deciding factor in weight lifting competitions such as the Bench Press, Squat, or Dead Lift. You know objectively that you are becoming stronger when you can lift more weight than you were able to lift previously. Such measurements, however, are not feasible or useful when you are trying to determine if you are increasing the strength of your core muscles. The interrelated muscular movements of the lower torso and hips are too complex to be measured by lifts in a single plane of motion, such as the three competitive events listed above.

If you cannot determine objectively whether your core strength is improving by the amount of weight you can lift, how can you know if you are making progress? The answer is simple. As with "strength," you employ a <u>functional</u> definition of "stronger" to measure your progress. Is this subjective? Yes, but also very useful.

You can utilize the skills, knowledge, and bodily awareness you have developed by training your core muscles in the gym and apply these enhanced experiences to all other physical activities of your life. How? Pay attention to how your core muscles feel when you walk, when you pick up a heavy object, when you climb up a ladder, when you swing a golf club, or when you do hundreds of other physical activities every day. You <u>know</u> your core muscles are stronger because they feel stronger. The middle of your body feels more flexible. You can turn your torso with ease, just as you did a decade or two ago. You can pick up your grandchild and not feel as though your back might give out or that you will cause a hernia. The movements in your hips feel freer. You get in and out of your car easily. You walk up and down stairs with confidence, not one step at a time. In short, you feel as though your entire lower torso/hip complex is the smooth-moving center of your personal universe. In your youth, you took this feeling for granted, never were even conscious of it. Now, as a revitalized adult, you are highly aware of and extremely grateful for the leaner and stronger muscles around your equator. You do not need a scale or a tape measure to determine if you are stronger. You feel it way down deep in your core.

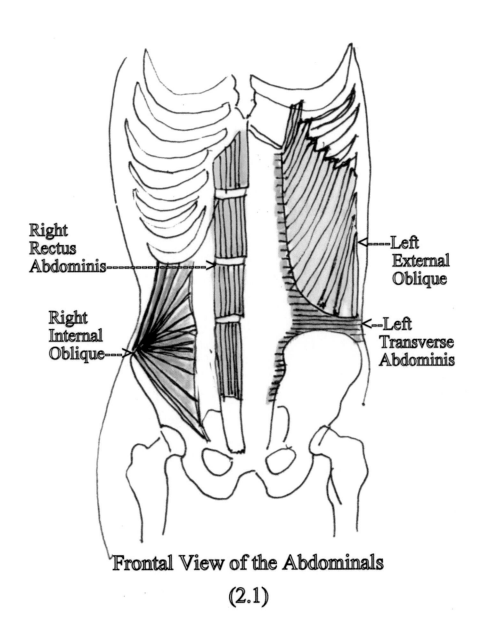

Frontal View of the Abdominals

(2.1)

Chapter 2

Why Not Strength for Life®?

Why "After 40"?

The subtitle of this book is "A Leaner Stronger Core After 40, After 65, and Beyond…" First of all, why do we single out age 40?

For centuries, human beings have grumbled about beginning to feel old as they approach and then reach forty years of age. Consider the opening quatrain of William Shakespeare's second sonnet:

> "When forty winters shall besiege thy brow
> And dig deep trenches in thy beauty's field,
> Thy youth's livery, so gazed on now,
> Will be a tattered weed, of small worth held."

Even into the 20th and 21st centuries, fear of age 40 has persisted. For many decades, the late comedian Jack Benny celebrated his 39th birthday every year. Today, most professional athletes are considered "over the hill" when they reach their 40th birthday, evidenced by the fact that the owners of their teams are no longer willing to offer them the same multiyear, multimillion-dollar contracts they had offered only a few years before. And it remains a tradition for our family members and friends to enjoy fiendish delight in throwing us surprise 40th birthday parties.

To be sure, some signs of physical deterioration that begin to appear around age 40 seduce us into believing the "40-is-getting-old" hypothesis. For many of us, reading a newspaper without glasses becomes problematic. And somewhere near our 40th birthday, we notice a little more hair accumulates on the drain cover after we take a shower. However, these are minor conditions of health over which we do not have much control. There are other, much more important, aspects of health over which we possess great potential for control. Most notably, we can avoid the accumulation of excess body fat, the tragic condition that plagues the majority of us who are American adults.

Between the ages of 25 and 55 years, an average American adult gradually gains more than 45 pounds of new body fat and loses about 15 pounds of lean body mass, primarily muscle and bone tissue. At 55, we weigh 30 pounds more than we did at age 25. But our real health deficit is 60 pounds—15 pounds less muscle to cart around 45 pounds more body fat. Chronologically, the exact center of this unfortunate age span is 40. Our blood pressure readings escalate. Type II diabetes sets in. Medication lists grow longer. Waistlines expand. Gradually, almost without realizing it, we lose the ability to participate in our favorite physical activities. We have allowed ourselves to become disabled prematurely. But let's reverse this.

Before you reach your 40th birthday, plan for it with great anticipation. Your goal is to have a great pattern of positive health habits firmly in place and already in action on the 40th anniversary of your birth. By learning to eat well, exercise intelligently, laugh a lot more and relax a little more, you will see age 40 as a diamond opportunity to become *leaner for life*, to enjoy great health, and to participate vigorously in your favorite physical activities for many decades to come.

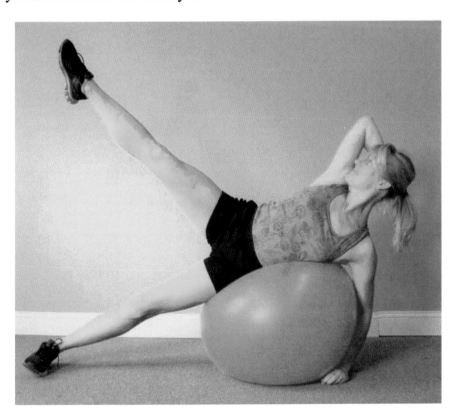

Why "After 65"?

If reaching 40 years of age is a time when some of us fall for the "I-am-feeling-old-and-achy" line of malarkey, arriving at the plateau of 65 years is when even more of us line up to order an "I-had-better-slow-down-now" baloney sandwich. Indeed, we do face some new health challenges during our second half century of life. And, yes, we do have to make some changes in the physical activities of our lives. But slowing down to a crawl and eating soft foods are not two of those changes. On the contrary, reaching 65 is a very loud call to action. For many health reasons, we need to eat more intelligently and to exert ourselves physically more often than we did in our previous six and one-half decades.

In general, the three-decade span from 25 to 55 years of age is when most of us gain massive amounts of excess body weight. Then, somewhere between ages 55 and 65, the average body weight of American adults begins to level off. After 65, most of us actually begin to lose body weight. Unfortunately, most of the body weight we lose after age 65 is lean body mass, primarily muscle and bone—the very tissues we need to maintain great posture and to perform the physical activities of life that are most important to us. In other words, we become weaker. Excessive loss of bone tissue is termed *osteoporosis*. Excessive loss of muscle tissue is known as *sarcopenia*. Together, these diseases of disuse rob of us of our strength. Not one of us can afford to sit by passively and permit these destructive processes to steal our vitality. Retirement schmirement! To the greatest extent of our individual potentials, we owe it to ourselves and to our loved ones to build and maintain our ***strength for life***!

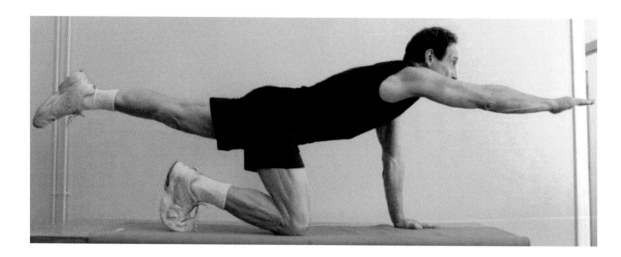

"and Beyond…"

70? 80? 90? You must be joking!

Not me.

Personally, I can only attest that we human beings can develop leaner and stronger core muscles after age 70. But, until you do your best to eat very well, to exercise intelligently, and to smile a lot every day, you do not know for how long in your life you can enjoy the freedom of good health. Give clean and active living your best shot! Maximize your personal potential for a long and lean, fruitful and meaningful, joyful and independent life. Go for it!

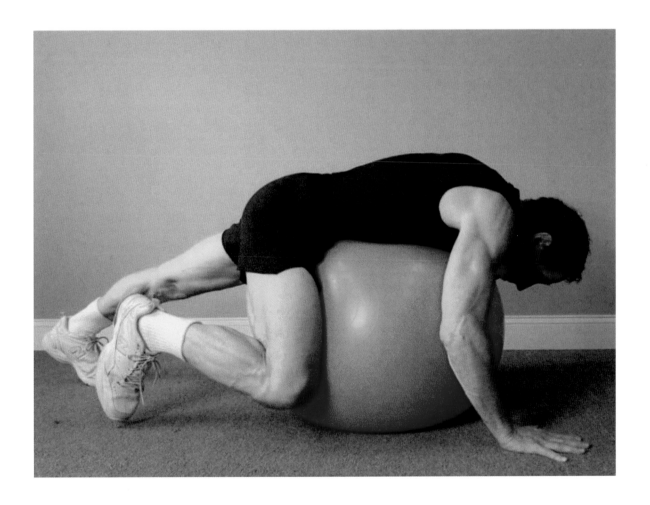

Chapter 3

Meet Your Abdominals and their Sidekicks

Without question, the abdominal muscles are the superstars of the lower torso/hip complex. Therefore, an effective core exercise program begins when you develop pictures in your mind of the locations and actions of the abdominals.

The abdominals are composed of four distinct muscle groups: (1) Rectus Abdominis, which causes your shoulders and upper torso to bend forward toward the knees; (2) External and (3) Internal Obliques, which cause your torso to turn and/or bend to each side; and (4) Transverse Abdominis, which can make your abdomen flatter by pulling it inward and slightly upward. Each of these four groups consists of two nearly identical muscles, one on the left side and one on the right, which attach to fibrous connective tissue near the center of the abdomen. In the illustration below, only the left external oblique and the right internal oblique are shown in order to visualize the directions in which the fibers of these muscles run.

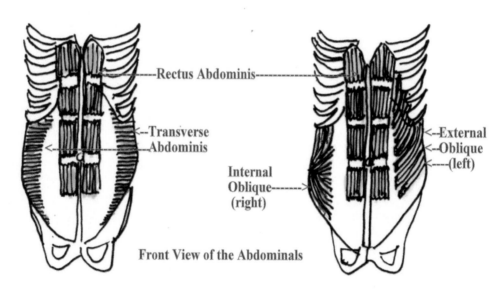

Front View of the Abdominals

e

Rectus Abdominis

The left and right rectus muscles run down the center of the torso from the bottom of your sternum to the pubic bone. The upper recti, above your navel, are the most superficial abdominals, their contours often visible on a lean person. As the upper recti contract, your shoulders and chest curl forward toward your lower torso.

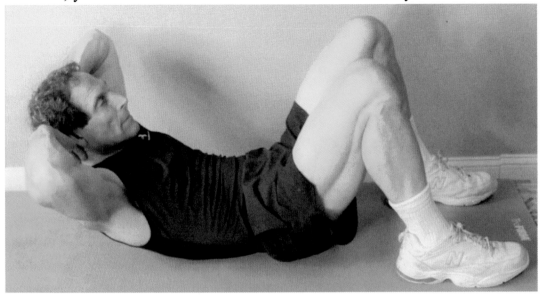

By contrast, when you contract your lower rectus muscles, located below your navel, you cause your lower torso to curl toward your chest and shoulders.

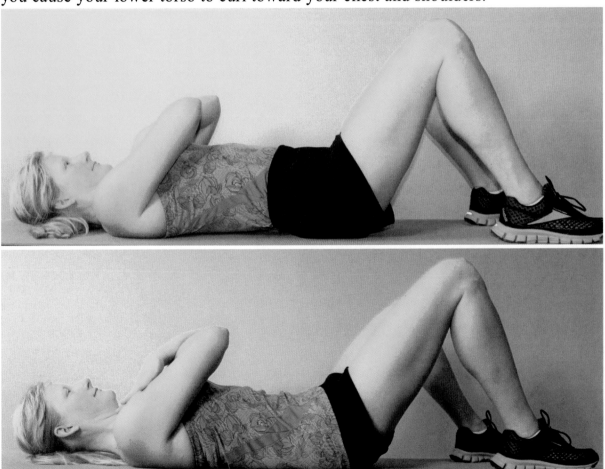

External Obliques
(Illustration 3.6)

The second most superficial of the abdominal muscles are the segmented right (shown in **3.6** below) and left external obliques. The muscle fibers of the upper segments of the external obliques run downward and diagonally from the front and sides of the lower ribs on each side and toward the center of the abdomen. At that point, the red muscle fibers end, but their tendons continue to form the abdominal aponeurosis, a flat fibrous membrane in the center of the abdomen. When your abdominal muscles are strong, the aponeurosis assists in holding your abdomen upward and backward toward the spine, promoting good posture. Conversely, when your abdominals are weak, the aponeurosis loses its retaining function and your belly sags forward, outward, and downward. The muscle fibers in the lower segments of the left and right external obliques, located more laterally, run downward from the sides of your lower ribs and attach to the top of the iliac crests.

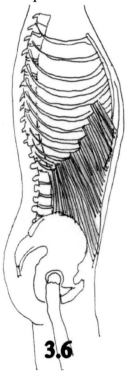

3.6

The external obliques play important roles in many human actions. When your left and right external obliques contract simultaneously, they assist the rectus abdominis in flexing your shoulders and chest toward the groin (**3.7**). When only the right external oblique contracts, your torso flexes forward and rotates to the left (**3.8**). When primarily the lateral and lower fibers of the right external oblique contract, they cause the torso to bend to that side (**3.9**). In short, the external obliques have many different actions. They require several different exercises, if you want to reach your potential to execute with ease and grace the physical acts of your daily life.

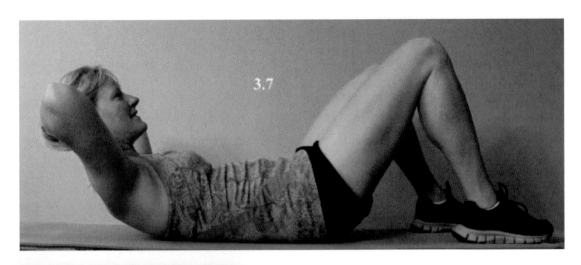

3.7

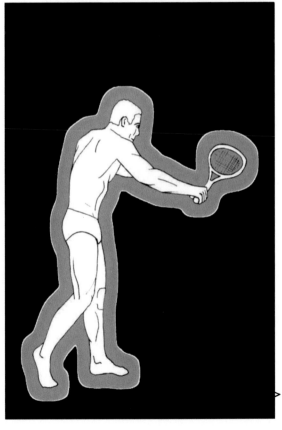

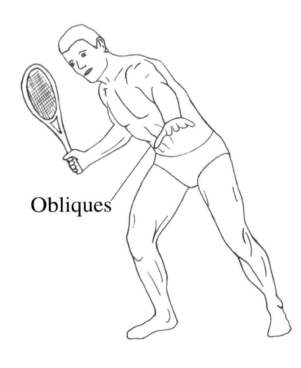

Obliques

Internal Obliques
(Illustration 3.10)

The internal obliques **(a)** are the next deepest layer of the abdominal muscles. The lower and middle internal oblique fibers run in opposing directions to the more superficial external obliques. Beginning near the groin **(b)** and front of the ilium **(c)**, these fibers run upward, where they attach to the lower ribs **(d),** and centrally, where they join the abdominal aponeurosis **(e).** Unlike the lower and middle fibers, the lateral fibers of the internal obliques run in the same direction as the lateral fibers of the external obliques. When the lateral internal and external obliques contract simultaneously on one side, they bend your torso to that side (**Illustration 3.9**).

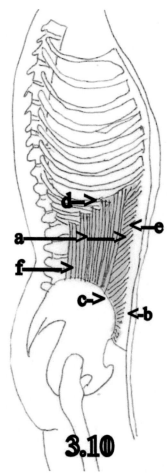

3.10

Like the external obliques, when both the right and left internal obliques contract simultaneously, they assist rectus abdominis in flexing the chest toward the groin and the groin toward the chest (**3.11**).

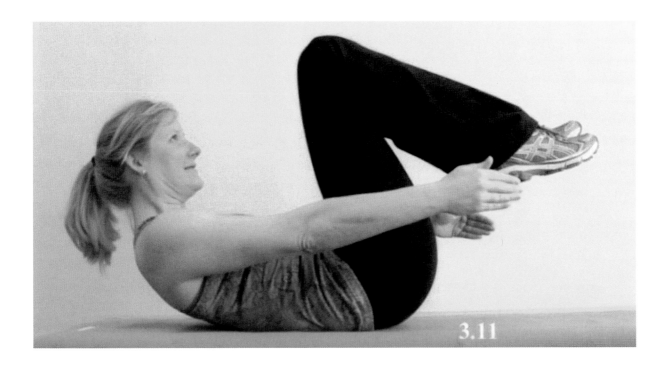

Because they actuate many diverse muscular functions in your core, the internal obliques should be challenged in several different exercises. For example, in the abdominal vacuum exercise pictured below, they assist transverse abdominis in compressing the abdomen (**3.12-3.13**).

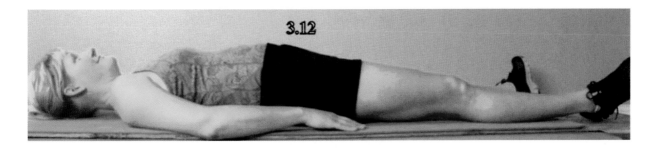

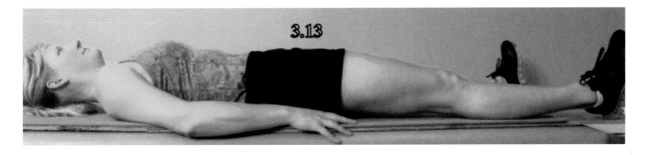

Transverse Abdominis
(Illustration 3.14)

The right **(3.14a)** and left transverse abdomini are the deepest of the abdominal muscles and have the simplest action. The fibers originate in: the lower rib cage (**b**); the lumbodorsal aponeurosis from the lower back (**c**); and from the front of the ilium and the inguinal area of the groin (**d**). The tendinous extensions of these fibers run centrally to join the abdominal aponeurosis (**e**) and then to the linea alba and the pubic bone (not shown here). The transverse abdominis has one important function—it "hollows" the abdomen, that is, pulls it inward and upward (**3.12 and 3.13**). Because its actions are limited, only one or two exercises are necessary to develop full strength. However, once you master the action of this muscle, you can incorporate it as an essential element in nearly every other abdominal exercise.

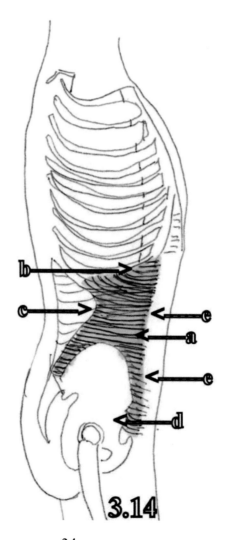

3.14

The Supporting Cast of the Core: Muscles of the Hips and Back

Although the "Abs" are the rock stars, the muscles of the hips and lower back are also important members of the "core." The more you concentrate upon how your muscles feel during each repetition of every exercise, the more aware you will become of how deeply interrelated these muscles are in hundreds of the physical acts you perform every day. Therefore, just as we did with the abdominal groups, we will review briefly the locations and actions of the hip and lower back muscles.

Hip Flexors

As the hip flexor muscles (most importantly iliopsoas and rectus femoris) contract, they cause the femur (thigh bone) to move forward and upward. Every time you lift a knee up and forward to walk, run, march, or to ascend stairs, these hip flexors are the prime movers.

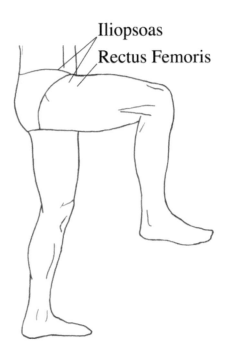

Iliopsoas
Rectus Femoris

In Illustrations **3.18** and **3.19**, the right iliopsoas and the right rectus femoris are shown in frontal views.

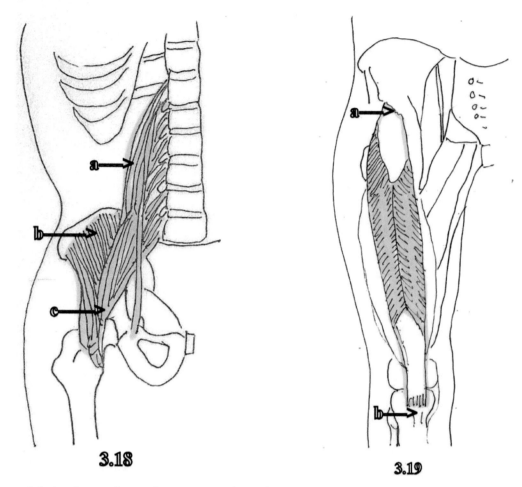

3.18   **3.19**

The iliopsoas (**c**) is the union of two muscles, the psoas (**a**) and the iliacus (**b**). The right and left psoas major muscles originate on the lateral aspects of the 12th thoracic vertebra and all five lumbar vertebrae. As shown in Illustration **3.18**, the right psoas muscle runs down from the spine and into the pelvic cavity where it joins iliacus to form the iliopsoas. The iliopsoas then continues southward until it attaches to the inside of the upper femur (upper leg bone).

Rectus femoris (**3.19**) is the longest of the quadriceps muscles and the only one that crosses the hip joint. In this frontal view of the right hip, we see rectus femoris originating on the front of the ilium (**a**) and running downward to the knee where it joins the patellar ligament to attach on the top and front of the tibia (**b**).

In addition to contributing to the iliopsoas muscles and to hip flexion, the psoas portions of iliopsoas can contract independently and in unison, causing extension of the lumbar spine. If this movement is sudden, violent, excessive, or repetitious, it may cause a jamming type of injury to the joints and supporting structures of the lower back. This is a major reason why the old-fashioned sit-up exercise often caused lower back injuries. However, this potential injury can be prevented by performing abdominal exercises with the spine pressed firmly to the floor due to continuous powerful contractions of the lower rectus abdominis (**3.15-3.17**).

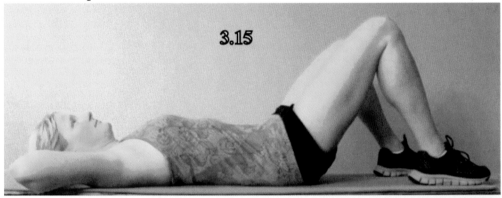

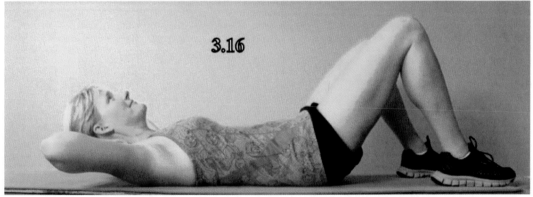

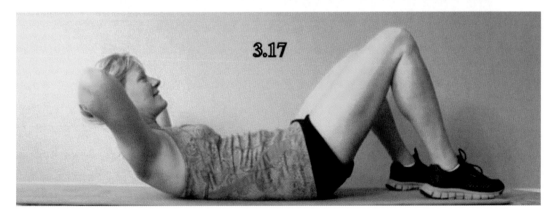

When both iliopsoas muscles contract at the same time, the result is flexion of both hips and a stretching of the extensor muscles of the lower back. This shown below in the Hanging Double Bent Knee Raise (**Illustrations 3.20-3.21**).

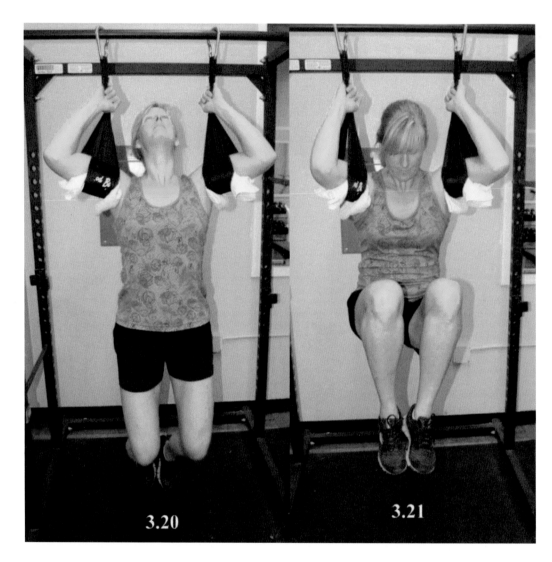

Because the rectus femoris crosses two joints, both the hip and the knee, it has two primary actions which can occur simultaneously or independently. Contraction of this muscle causes flexion of the hip and/or extension of the knee. With regard to abdominal strengthening, we need to be aware of rectus femoris as we perform any exercise that requires hip flexion (**Illustration 3.22**).

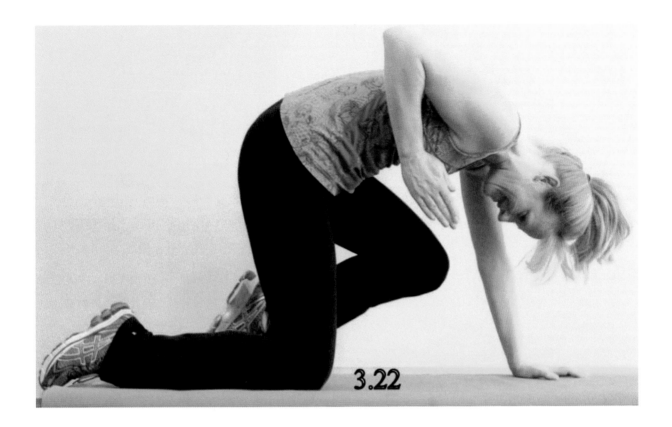

3.22

In addition to their roles in movement of the hip, the hip flexors can influence our abdominals in another way. If these muscles lose their flexibility, they tend to shorten over time and contribute to a forward leaning posture. Such a miscarriage throws the human body out of balance, expediting the development of the lower abdominal paunch as well as an upper thoracic kyphosis, excessive forward rounding of the upper back.

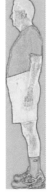

Clearly, the hip flexors are essential core muscles. As we will see next, the extensors of our hips are equally important members of our core.

Hip Extensors

The primary hip extensor muscles are the gluteus maximus and the hamstrings. In **Illustration 3.23**, a rear view of the right hip, we see how the right gluteus maximus originates on the sacrum and the back of the iliac crest and then runs laterally and downward to attach on the back of the femur. Your gluteus maximus, when well-conditioned, enables you to extend your hips powerfully as you move your body forward (**Illustration 3.24**). In addition, your glutes play a major role in holding you upright, even when you are standing still. They have a profound influence upon your posture, whether you are in motion or stationery. As well, a strong pair of glutes serves as a perfect counterbalance to strong abdominals. On the other hand, if a person's gluteal muscles become weak, the rear end sags, the pelvis rolls backward and downward, and your lower abdomen will protrude (bottom of page 39).

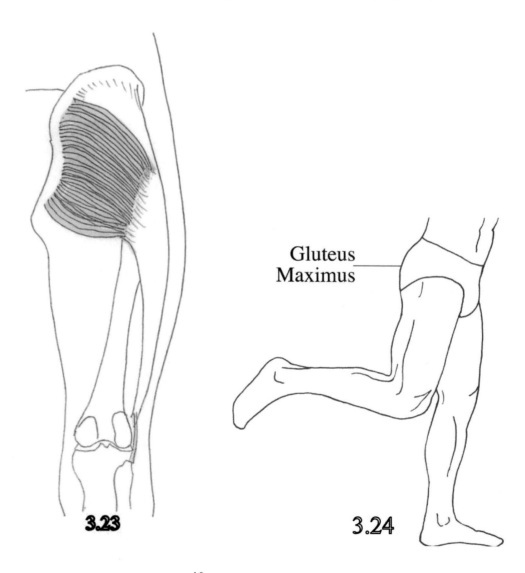

Gluteus
Maximus

3.23   3.24

Hip Extensors and Flexors of the Knee: Hamstrings

Illustration 3.25 is another rear view of the right hip, but with the more superficial gluteals removed. Thus, we see the right hamstring muscles, which originate on the lower aspect of the ischium and run downward to attach on the back of the femur and then to the back of the lower leg bones, the tibia and fibula. All three of the hamstring muscles cross both the hip and the knee joints, meaning both that they cause flexion of the knee (**3.26**) and that they assist gluteus maximus in extension of the hip (**3.27**). If our hamstring muscles lose their flexibility, they tend to cause poor posture and lower back pain, as well as make it difficult or risky to perform some advanced abdominal exercises. Therefore, the hamstrings are essential members of the core.

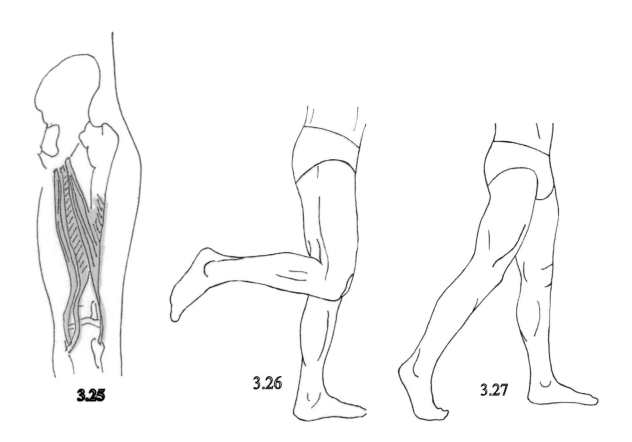

3.25   3.26   3.27

Hip Abductors

In two rear views of the right hip below, we see gluteus medius (**3.28**) and, underneath it, gluteus minimus (**3.29**). In the side view of the right hip (**3.30**), we see tensor fascia lata, a small muscle that would be covered by your holster if you were an Old Wild West gunslinger. These three muscles join a long tendon running down the side of your leg to just below your knee (picture below). They are prime movers in abducting the hip and in stabilizing us laterally when we are standing, walking, running, and even when we are on "all fours". We must keep them strong and flexible to maintain good posture and balance as we age. In **Illustration 3.31**, the right abductors do the unsung job of stabilizing the right hip while the abductors on the left grab the glory by moving the left leg out to the side.

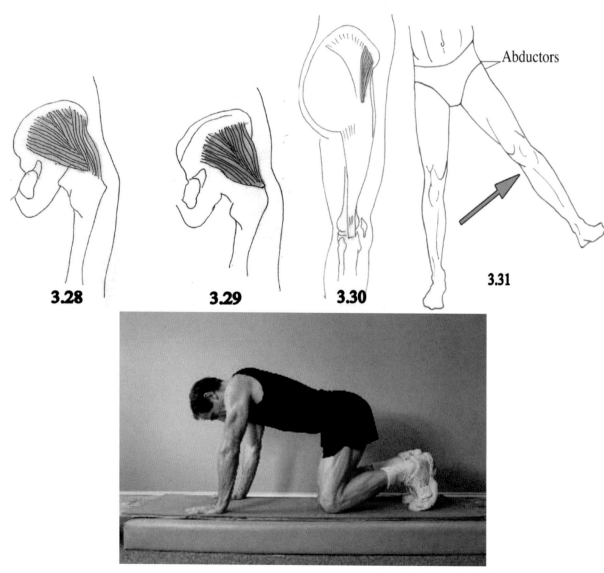

External Rotators of the Hip

Illustration 3.32 is a rear view of the external rotators of the right hip. When these muscles contract, they rotate the upper leg outward. You use the muscles each time you turn your leg and hips outward to exit from of a car, or when you pivot your back leg to hit a forehand in tennis (**3.33**). In many acts of daily life, as well as in many exercises for the obliques, the external rotators work intimately with the hip abductors. These muscles also play critical roles in providing lateral stability as we walk, run, and stand. By including exercises to strengthen these muscles in your core strengthening program, you are increasing the value of your fitness investments.

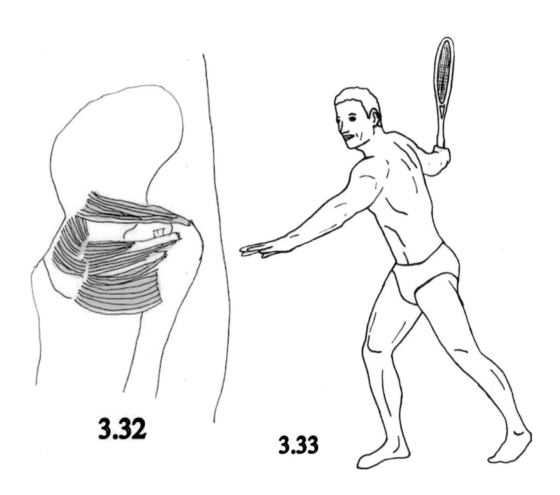

3.32

3.33

Hip Adductors/Internal Rotators

The hip adductor muscles are attached to the front of the pelvis at the pubic bone and then run laterally and downward to the medial and rear aspect of the femur (thigh bone). A front view of the right hip adductor group is shown in **Illustration 3.34**. Conversely, in **Illustration 3.35** we see the left adductors in action. As the left adductor muscles contract, they bring the upper leg from a position away from the side of the body back toward the center and slightly beyond, as in kicking a soccer ball. In addition to adduction of the hip, the adductors assist in other movements, such as internal rotation and flexion of the hip. They also work in concert with the internal obliques to hold us in the saddle when we ride horses, ostriches, and motorcycles.

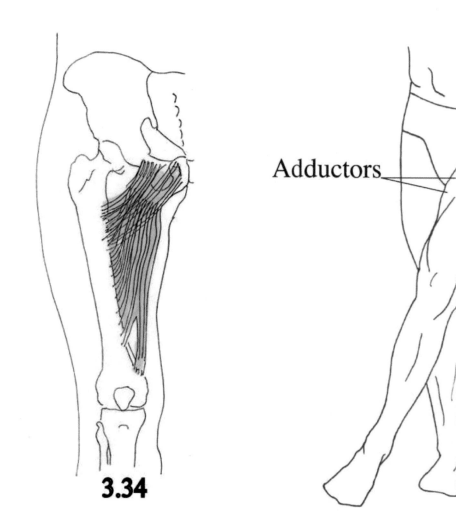

Adductors

3.34

3.35

There are many practical reasons why developing the entire core muscle complex is important. For instance, total core strength is essential to placing yourself in the optimal position from which to look for a lost contact lens.

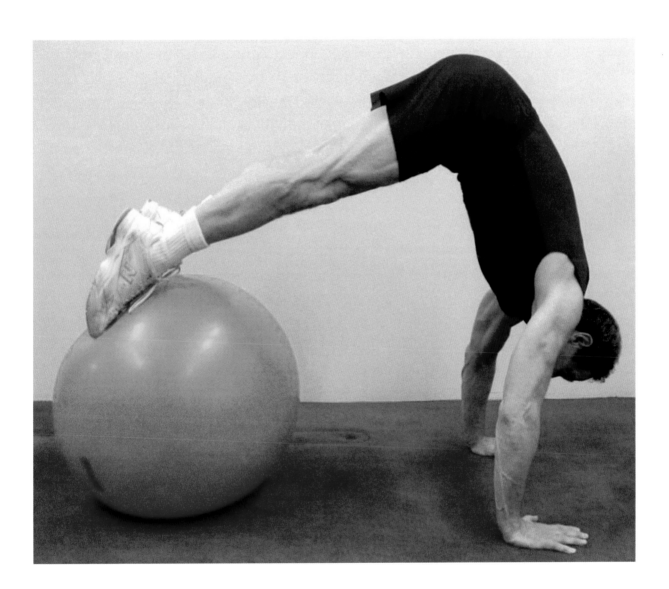

Spinal Muscles

It seems obvious that, if we work diligently to strengthen the front and sides of our lower torso/hip complex, we should also strengthen and improve the flexibility of the muscles in the lower back. This inspires us to think of our lower torso complex as a cylinder with overlapping muscles winding around our entire circumference and producing smooth controlled movements in all types of human activity. What may seem less obvious, however, is that we need to strengthen not just the lower back muscles, but all our spinal muscles, including those of the middle and upper back, and even those as far north as the top of the neck. Developing integrity in all these spinal muscles is essential to achieving and maintaining excellent posture as we age. In addition, the upper spinal muscles must be strong and flexible if we are to execute many abdominal exercises safely and effectively.

Illustration 3.36 is a rear view of the spine with the **erector spinae** muscles drawn in on the right side only (excepting one small muscle group added at the base of the skull on the left). The erector spinae are a magnificent complex of muscles running the up the entire spine, in a variety of directions and lengths, from the sacrum up to the base of the skull. As these spinal muscles ascend, some attach to one or more vertebrae above, while others fan out to attach to ribs. When the right and left members of the erector spinae contract simultaneously, they cause extension of the torso (**3.37**). When these muscles contract on only one side, they contribute to lateral bending of the torso to that side (**3.38**)

Continuing to build the strength and flexibility of your erector spinae is essential to <u>improving</u> your health and vitality as you age. Allowing these muscles to become weak, stiff, and flabby will diminish the integrity of your entire musculoskeletal structure and compromise the function of all other organ systems of your body. In addition, losing strength in your spinal muscles will cause you to slouch when you walk, to breathe shallowly, and to shuffle your feet. Stooping posture impairs digestion. Conversely, keeping these muscles strong and pliable will help you maintain erect posture, breathe freely and deeply, walk with majesty, digest food properly, and execute with grace all the other meaningful physical acts of your life.

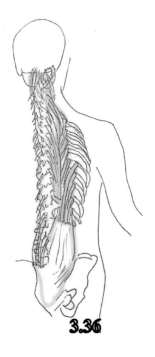

3.36

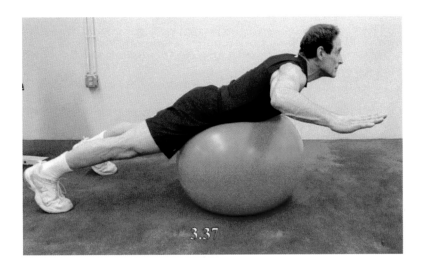

3.37

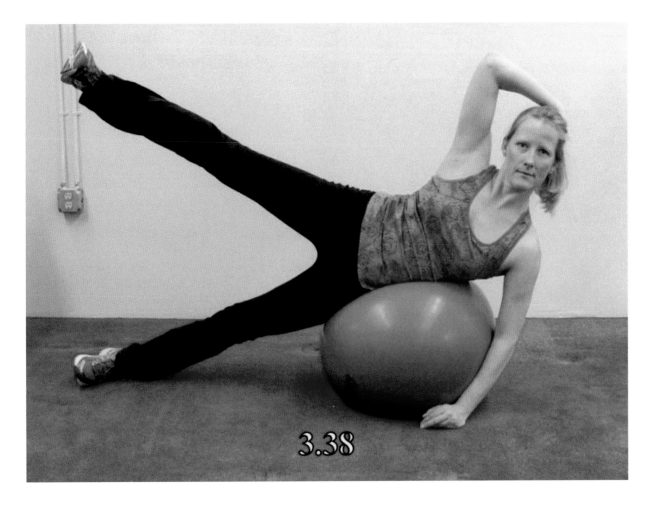

3.38

47

Illustration 3.39 is a rear view of the lower back and pelvis. A few inches to each side of the spine in the lower back, the **quadratus lumborum muscle** (only right illustrated here) originates on the crest of the ilium and rises to attach to the 12th rib and the transverse processes of the lumbar vertebrae. When the left and right quadratus muscles contract simultaneously, they assist in extension of the lower spine. When only one quadratus muscle contracts, it assists in lateral bending of the torso to that side and/or lifting the hip on that side (**3.40**).

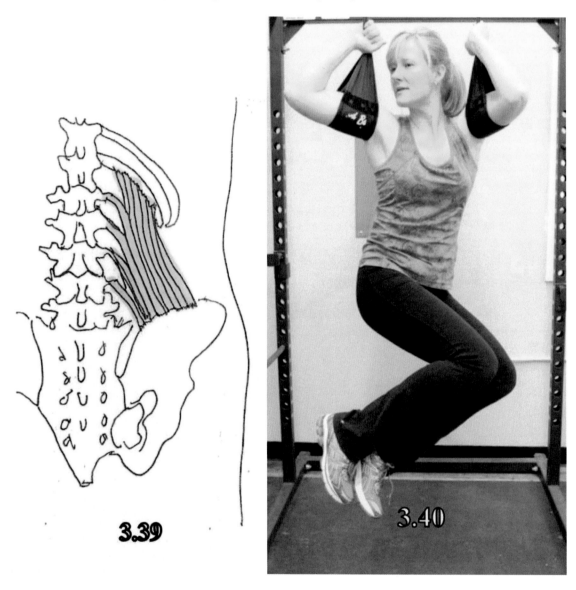

3.39

3.40

Smaller Spinal Muscles

Underneath the erector spinae and other longer, larger, and more superficial muscles of the back, are groups of smaller spinal muscles known collectively as the **transversospinalae**. These deep central spinal muscles are present up and down the entire spine. Most of these muscles span only two to six spinal levels. However, they are essential to the smooth execution in all the intricate and coordinated movements we expect our bodies to be able to do. If you execute lower torso exercises with precision and care, you increase the strength and flexibility of these vital muscle groups. When the members on both sides contract simultaneously, they assist in extension of the vertebral column. When only the muscles on one side contract, they contribute to lateral flexion and/or rotation of the spine. These muscles are too small and too numerous to picture in your mind as you perform exercises for the lower torso/hip complex. However, it is instructive to know that they are there and that you are strengthening them when you do core exercises. These muscles are small but important contributors to the integrity in your entire musculoskeletal system. **Illustration 3.41** is a drawing of three spinal levels from the rear and demonstrates three of these small spinal muscles groups, **rotatores (a)**, **interspinales (b)**, and **intertransversarii (c)**.

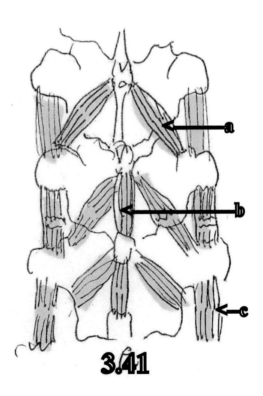

3.41

In the upper back and posterior neck regions, most of the deep spinal muscles are higher versions of the **erector spinae** and **transversospinalae** of the lower and middle back. However, superficial to these deep spinal muscles are two other important muscle groups of the neck. **Illustration 3.42** is a rear view of the upper spine showing the **right splenius capitis (a)** and the **left splenius cervicis (b)** muscles. These posterior upper spinal muscles enhance our ability to extend, rotate, and laterally flex the neck and upper thorax, movements which occur repeatedly as we perform exercises for the lower torso/hip complex. Strength and flexibility in all muscles of the neck are critical to the successful performance of most physical activities. Many exercises for your core cannot be performed safely or effectively if your neck is weak or stiff. Thus, I urge you to study *Neck Strength for Life®,* which I have written as a companion text to the Abdominal Strength for Life® program.

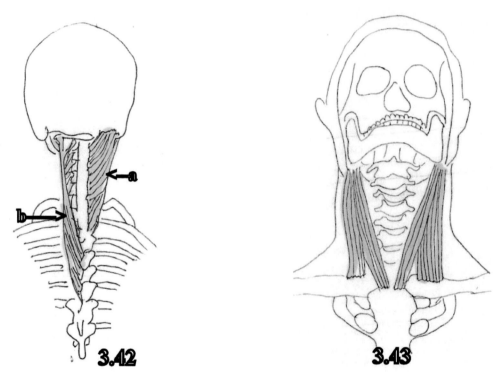

In **Illustration 3.43**, a frontal view of the neck, we see the right and left **sternocleidomastoideus** (SCM) muscles. When the SCMs on both sides contract simultaneously, they enable you to flex your head and neck forward. When only one side contracts, they facilitate lateral flexion and rotation of your head . Therefore, these muscles are involved in nearly every abdominal exercise—**Illustration 3.44**, for example—and must be strong and and flexible if we are to perform core exercises effectively and without injuring ourselves.

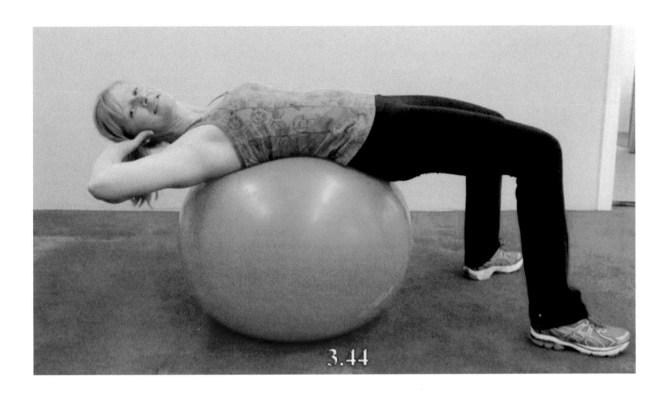

3.44

In addition to the deeper upper spinal muscles, at least three other, more superficial, upper spinal muscles affect our posture profoundly. In **Illustration 3.45**, the left **trapezius (a)**, right **rhomboids (b)**, right **levator scapulae (c)** are shown. Developing these muscles helps to prevent CHD (computer hump disorder). For this reason, a few simple exercises to keep these muscles strong are included in the Abdominal Strength for Life® Program (**Illustration 3.46**).

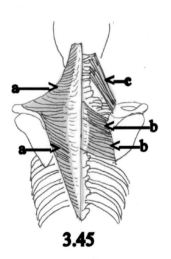

3.45

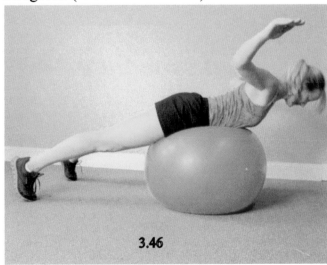

3.46

Part II

The Abdominal Strength for Life® Program: Beginning and Intermediate Levels

Chapter 4   *Beginning Level*
                     Abdominal Medley#1

Chapter 5   *Intermediate Level*
                     Abdominal Medley #2

Chapter 6   *Intermediate Level*
                     Abdominal Medley #3

Fundamentals of Core Exercise Execution

1. Every repetition of every core muscle exercise has **two distinct phases**.

    a. Contraction Phase: From a fully stretched Beginning Position, contract your target muscles slowly as you initiate and then continue movement to an intensely contracted Peak Position. Pause briefly.

    b. Extension Phase: From the fully contracted Peak Position, return slowly to the fully stretched Beginning Position. Pause briefly.

2. Pause momentarily at the end of each phase.

The pause at the end of each phase provides an instant to focus upon contracting or extending your target muscles for the upcoming phase. In the contraction phase, because you must overcome inertia, initiating movement from a complete stop requires more muscular energy and builds more strength than bouncing from repetition to repetition. Ten repetitions with a pause at the end of each phase are superior to one hundred done with herky-jerky haste.

3. Focus intently as you contract and then lengthen your target muscles throughout every millimeter of movement of every repetition. Strive constantly to feel these movements in your target muscles.

4. The breathing pattern for every exercise is identical.

    a. Exhale throughout the Contraction Phase. Inhale throughout Extension Phase.

    b. In the Beginning Position, before you begin movement, inhale.

    c. As you start the Contraction Phase, begin to exhale. Exhaling as you compress your thorax prevents a Valsalva Maneuver, which can temporarily block blood and oxygen flow to your heart.

    d. Continue to exhale slowly throughout the Contraction Phase.

    e. Pause momentarily in the Peak Position.

    f. As you initiate the Extension Phase, begin to inhale.

    g. Continue to inhale slowly until you reach the Beginning Position.

    h. When you breathe in this manner, the rate of your bodily movements becomes synchronous with your rate of breathing, Slow and steady movement is ideal for developing strength in your core muscles.

Chapter 4

Abdominal Medley # 1

The Beginning Level

Abdominal Medley #1 is an introduction to the building blocks of superb core muscle strength and flexibility. Once you master these six fundamental exercises, you can intensify your training dramatically by performing more complex variations in Intermediate Level Medleys #2 and #3.

As described on the previous page, in "Fundamentals of Core Exercise Execution," you must strive to perform all exercises in Abdominal Medley #1 slowly, through relatively full ranges of motion, with precision, and with great mental focus. If you strive for these qualities of execution, you will be amazed at how quickly you increase the strength and flexibility of all the muscle groups in your lower torso/hip complex.

After perusing Chapter 3, you have a rudimentary knowledge of the muscles of the lower torso/hip complex. You are beginning to develop a motion picture of these interrelated muscle groups in action. As you perform each repetition of each exercise, you feel and "see" your target muscles at work. When you reach this level of exercise consciousness, you are truly experiencing the thrill of physical exertion.

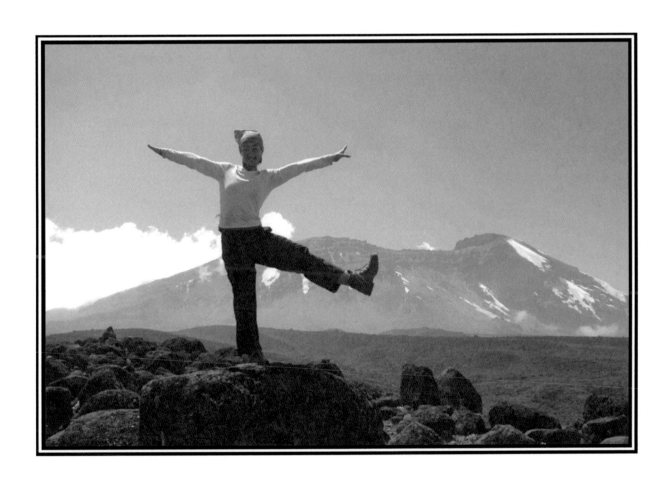

Abdominal Medley #1

1. Lower Abdominal Curl

a. Primary Target Muscle Group: Right and Left Lower Rectus Abdominis

b. This is the foundation for nearly all other abdominal exercises. Reaching and holding the lower rectus down position builds a compact and powerful lower abdominal musculature.

c. Directions

(1) Lie on your back with your knees bent and your feet flat on the floor. Cross your arms across your chest or rest your hands at your sides. As you inhale moderately through your nose, allow your lower spine and abdomen to arch upward slightly toward the ceiling (**Illustration 4.1**). Pause momentarily.

(2) As you begin to exhale, use your lower rectus abdominis muscles to push your lower back down firmly against the floor and rotate the front of your pelvis up toward your ribcage while keeping your sacrum and upper gluteals firmly against the floor (**Illustration 4.2**). This is **the lower rectus down position**, which you must maintain continuously throughout the performance of many other abdominal exercises. However, in this basic exercise you will hold the down position only for two seconds, until you exhale completely.

(3) As you begin to inhale, allow your lower rectus muscles to relax, which will cause your pelvis and the segments of your lower spine to return to their respective beginning positions (**4.1**). Pause momentarily.

(4) As you begin to exhale, repeat steps (2) and (3) for a total of 10 repetitions. Try to contract your lower rectus and push your lower spine down more firmly with each successive repetition.

(5) At the completion of the last repetition, maintain the lower rectus down position and proceed seamlessly to the next exercise of this abdominal medley. As in a relay race in competitive swimming, there is no break between each leg of the medley.

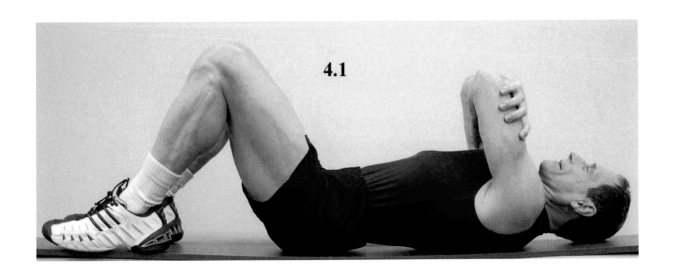

4.1

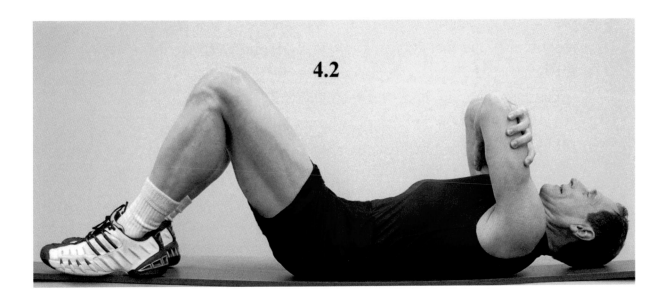

4.2

1 A. Single Bent Knee Raise

a. Primary Target Muscle Groups: Lower Rectus Abdominis and Hip Flexors

b. This is a training exercise only and not primarily for the abdominals. If you found the previous exercise easy to perform, skip over this one and move on the Upper Abdominal Curl. The present exercise is included here for anyone who finds it difficult to master the essential skill of maintaining the lower rectus down position continuously during the performance of a core exercise while in the supine recumbent position. In this case, the prime movers are the hip flexors, especially iliopsoas and rectus femoris.

c. Directions

    (1) Continuing in the lower rectus down position from the last repetition of the first exercise, inhale moderately (**Illustration 4.3**).

    (2) As you exhale, raise your right knee until it is directly over your waistline. Maintain the lower rectus down position continuously (**Illustration 4.4**). Hold this position momentarily.

    (3) Try not to alter the 90°degree bend in your right knee.

    (4) As you inhale, lower your right foot to the beginning position, always using your lower rectus abdominis to keep your lower back pressed tightly to the floor (**Illustration 4.3**).

    (5) Pause momentarily, then exhale as you repeat steps (2) to (4).

    (6) Do 10 to 15 repetitions on each side. Once this exercise becomes easy to perform, omit it from your workout routine.

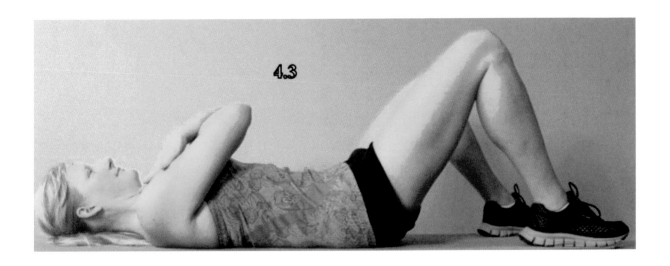

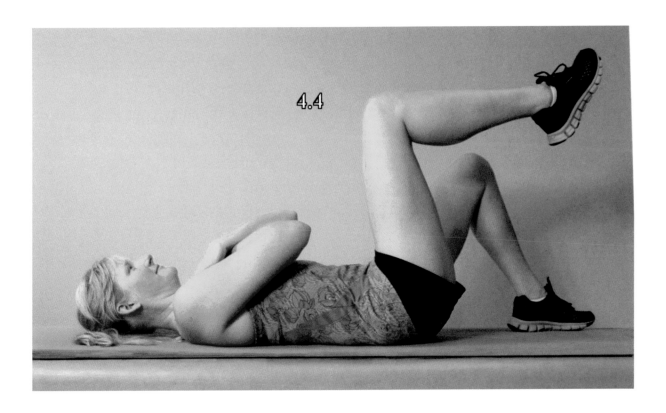

2. Upper Abdominal Curl

a. Primary Target Muscle Group: Upper Rectus Abdominis
Secondary Target Muscle Group: Lower Rectus Abdominis
b. This is the quintessential abdominal exercise. If we perform it with precision, concentration, and in a continuous lower rectus down position, we can realize tremendous benefits. As you can see in **Illustration 4.7** below, the word "curl" describes accurately the curling and uncurling actions of the torso, head, and shoulders as the upper rectus abdominis muscles contract powerfully in this exercise.

c. Directions

(1) Start in the lower rectus down position with your fingers lightly supporting your neck (**Illustration 4.5**). Inhale moderately.

(2) Begin to exhale as you curl first your head, then your chest and shoulders, slowly and smoothly toward your knees. **Illustration 4.6** is halfway up. Keep your elbows back, in the same plane as your ears, as pictured. Use your fingers only to support your neck gently and not to pull your head forward. Continue curling your chest and shoulders up and forward until your upper rectus abdominis feels very tightly contracted (**Illustration 4.7**). Your shoulder blades should be just off the mat. Hold this "up" position for one to two seconds.

(3) As you begin to inhale, uncurl your shoulders, chest, and head slowly back to the beginning position (**Illustration 4.5**), using your lower rectus abdominis to keep your lower back firmly against the floor throughout your descent.

(4) Pause momentarily and then repeat steps (2) and (3).

(5) Do 10 to 20 repetitions with great concentration. It is much more beneficial to do a limited number of repetitions intensely rather than dozens of repetitions with mental meandering.

(6) At the completion of the last repetition, maintain the lower rectus down position and glide directly into the next exercise of the medley.

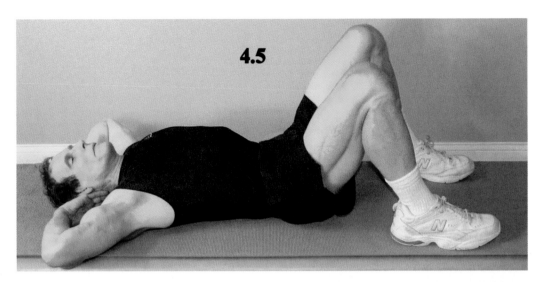

4.5

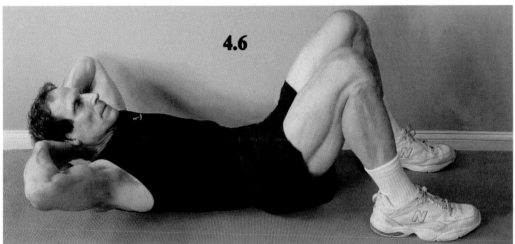

4.6

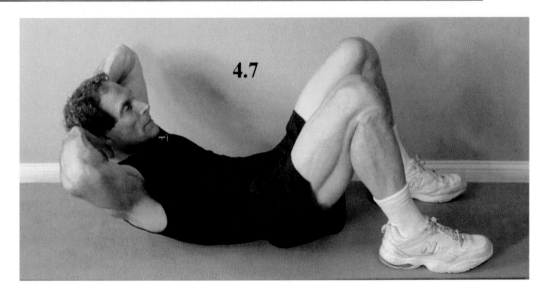

4.7

3. Diagonal Abdominal Curl

a. Primary Target Muscle Groups: External Obliques, Upper and Lower Rectus Abdominis

b. In this exercise we combine the straight upper abdominal curl with slow rotation of the torso.

c. Directions

(1) In the lower rectus down position, leave your right hand behind your neck and your right elbow near the mat. Your knees remain bent and your feet flat on the mat. Turn your head to the right and look at your elbow. Place your left hand on the floor to the side of your left hip. This is the beginning position of the right diagonal abdominal curl (**Illustration 4.8**). Inhale moderately.

(2) As you begin to exhale, curl your head, neck, and right shoulder upward and diagonally to the left. At the same time, raise your left knee upward and to the right (**Illustration 4.9**).

(3) Continue curling your right elbow toward your rising your left knee until your right external obliques and your upper and lower rectus abdominis feel very tightly and fully contracted (**Illustration 4.10**). Pause momentarily to focus upon how these muscles feel in their peak contraction positions.

(4) Throughout both the contraction and lengthening phases of this exercise, maintain continuously the lower rectus down position.

(5) As you begin to inhale, uncurl your target muscles as well as your neck, right shoulder, right elbow, and left knee slowly and smoothly back to the beginning position.

(6) When you reach the beginning position, pause momentarily but do not relax your lower rectus. Continue looking at your right elbow; pause to enjoy a great stretch in your right external oblique muscles.

(7) As you begin to exhale, repeat steps (2) through (6), but try to achieve slightly stronger contractions with each successive repetition.

(8) Do 10 to 15 repetitions on the right side and then 10 to 15 on the left, always maintaining a strong lower rectus down position.

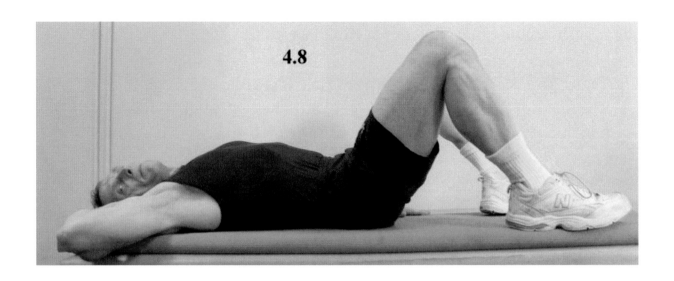

4.8

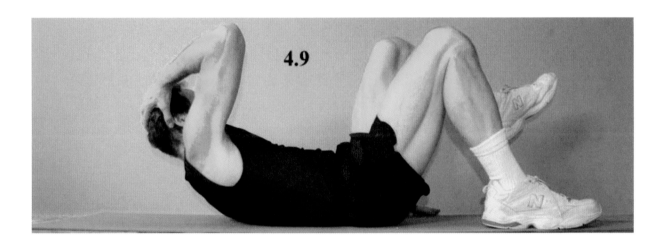

4.9

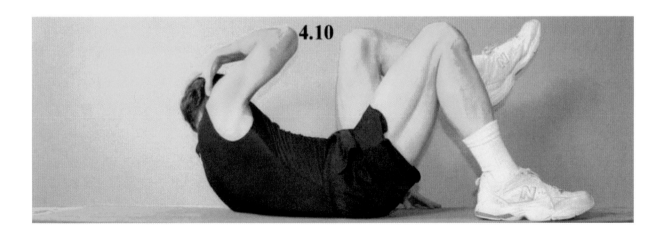

4.10

4. Abdominal Vacuum (aka: Abdominal Hollowing)

a. Target Muscle Group: Left and Right Transverse Abdominis

b. The fibers of these paired muscles run horizontally (**Sketch A**-side view), that is, at right angles to rectus abdominis (**Sketch B**-front view). They do not play a direct role in flexing your torso—curling your chest forward toward your pelvis or vice versa. Therefore, do not concern yourself with the lower rectus in this exercise. The major functions of the transverse abdomini are to depress or flatten the abdomen and to pull it inward and slightly upward.

c. Directions

(1) Lie flat on your back with your legs straight and hands at your sides.

(2) Inhale deeply and slowly as you allow all the abdominal muscles to relax as your abdomen rises like bread dough (**Illustration 4.11**).

(3) As you begin to exhale, contract your transverse abdomini to pull your abdomen inward toward your spine and upward slightly toward your sternum.

(4) Ideally, you should feel a hollowed-out depression extending from your pelvic region up to the lower tip of your sternum (**Illustration 4.12**).

(5) Maintain this hollowed out position for 2 seconds.

(6) As you begin to inhale slowly and deeply, allow your target muscles to relax and return to the beginning position (**Illustration 4.11**).

(7) Repeat steps (3) to (6) 10 times. With each successive repetition, endeavor to hollow out your abdomen a little more deeply.

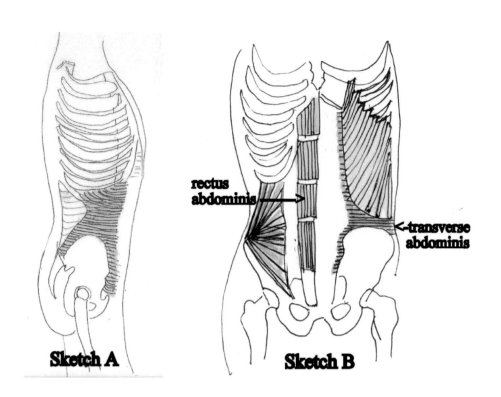

Sketch A

rectus abdominis

<-transverse abdominis

Sketch B

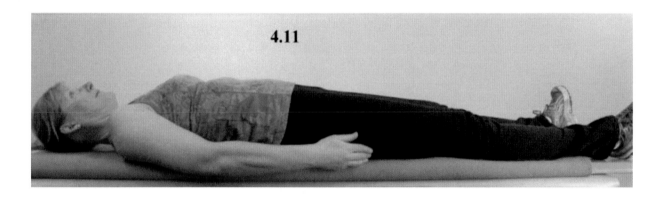

4.11

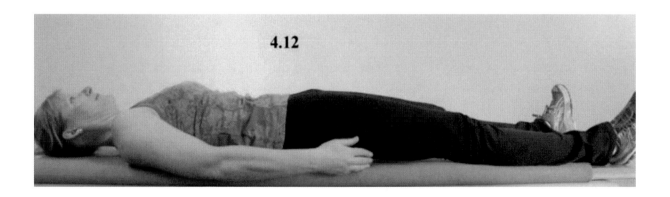

4.12

5A. Side Curl

a. Target Muscle Groups: External and Internal Obliques

b. This exercise stimulates the lateral fibers of your oblique muscles, which on each side run between the lower ribs and the crest of the ilium.

c. Directions

(1) Lie on your left side with your knees touching. The palm of your right hand is on top of your head with your fingertips just touching the top of your left ear which, in turn, should be touching or nearly touching the floor. The fingertips of your left hand should be resting on your right lower torso, just above the iliac crest (**Illustration 4.13**). This is the beginning position. Inhale moderately.

(2) As you begin to exhale, raise your head and left shoulder from the floor as you move your right elbow in an arcing motion upward, toward the ceiling. **Illustration 4.14** is the halfway point. With the fingertips of your left hand, you will feel a tightening of the oblique muscles on your right side.

(3) When you reach the highest point, where it feels as though the obliques are fully contracted (**Illustration 4.15**), pause momentarily to enjoy this sensation.

(4) Inhale as you lower your head and left shoulder slowly back to their beginning positions. With your left fingertips you will feel a pleasant stretch in your right obliques. This is a great example of how most strength training exercises are also flexibility exercises—if we perform them through full ranges of motion. Here the objective is not primarily to touch one's left ear to the floor; rather, it is to feel a moderate stretch in the right lateral obliques.

(5) Repeat steps (2) to (4) as you perform 10 to 15 concentrated repetitions while lying on your left side and then do the same while lying on your right side.

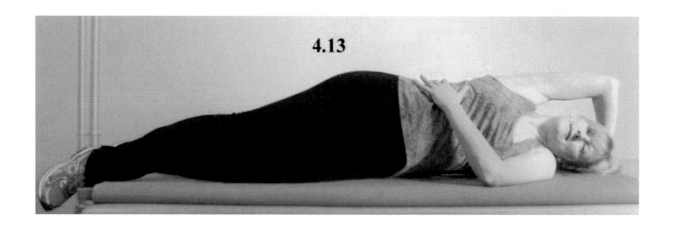

4.13

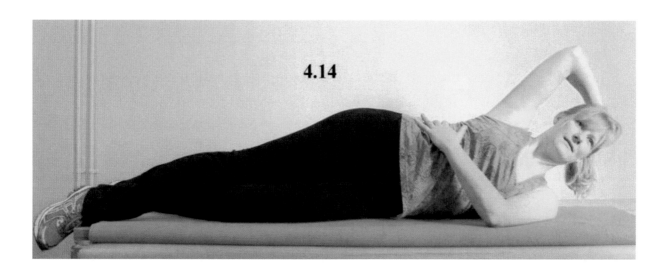

4.14

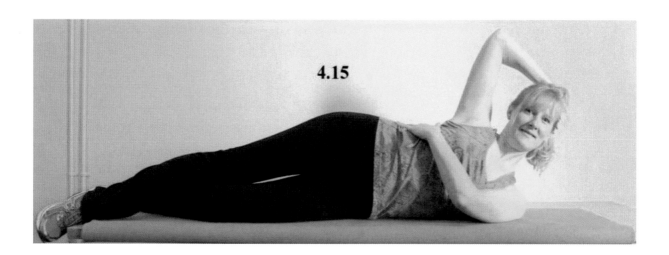

4.15

5B. Side Leg Raise

a. Target Muscles: Hip Abductors—primarily Gluteus Medius, Gluteus Minimus, and Tensor Fascia Lata.

b. This is not an abdominal exercise. However, it does build strength and flexibility in our adjacent hip muscles. As stated before, abdominal muscles do not exist in isolation. In most human movements, the abdominal muscles work in concert with other muscle groups, particularly of the hips, making it imperative that we address these related core muscle groups. Such a training philosophy helps us to become more balanced, agile, and fully developed physical human beings.

c. Directions

(1) Lie on your left side in the same beginning position as the side curl—with two slight alterations. Position your left arm on the floor in front of your torso. Move your bottom leg and foot forward about six inches, enough that the great toe of your right foot touches the floor just behind the heel of your left foot. This increases the stretch you will feel in your right hip abductor muscles. This is the beginning position (**Illustration 4.16**). Inhale.

(2) As you begin to exhale, raise your right leg and foot slowly toward the ceiling, trying to keep your right knee straight as you do. You will feel gradually increasing tightness in the target muscles on the outside of your right hip. Pause momentarily in the peak position when these muscles feel fully contracted (**Illustration 4.17**).

(3) As you begin to inhale, lower your right leg slowly to the beginning position. Enjoy the feeling of a great stretch in the target muscles as your right shoe touches the floor just behind the left heel.

(4) Do 10 to 15 repetitions while lying on your left side and then repeat while lying on your right side.

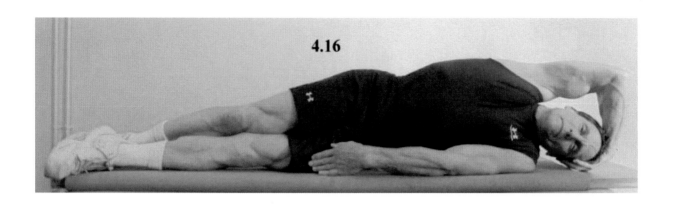

4.16

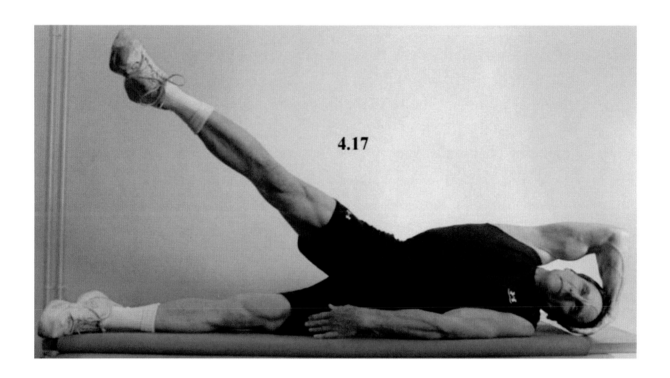

4.17

5. Side Jackknife

a. Target Muscles: Lateral Fibers of the External and Internal Obliques; Gluteus Medius and Minimus; and Tensor Fascia Lata.

b. Now that we have mastered the two previous exercises, we can save time by performing them simultaneously. The Side Curl and Side Leg Raise are merely the two halves of the Side Jackknife. However, it is worthwhile to learn the two previous exercises separately at first; this allows us to master important subtleties that we might miss if we start directly with the Side Jackknife.

c. Directions

(1) Lie on your left side with the fingertips of your right hand touching the top of your left ear. Your left arm rests on the floor in front of your torso. The medial portion of your right shoe touches the floor just behind the heel of your left shoe. **Illustration 4.18** is the beginning position. Inhale.

(2) As you begin to exhale, simultaneously: lift your head and left shoulder from the floor; move your right elbow in an arcing motion upward and toward your right hip; and lift your right leg and foot toward the ceiling (**Illustration 4.19**).

(3) When you reach the peak position, in which your right oblique and right hip abductor muscles feel fully contracted, pause momentarily (**Illustration 4.20**).

(4) Begin to inhale as you lower your right leg and left shoulder back toward their starting positions. When you reach the beginning position, pause momentarily to feel a great stretch in your target muscles before beginning to exhale as you start the next repetition.

(5) Repeat steps (2)-(4) for 10 to 15 concentrated repetitions while lying on your left side. Then perform the same number of thoughtful repetitions while on your right side.

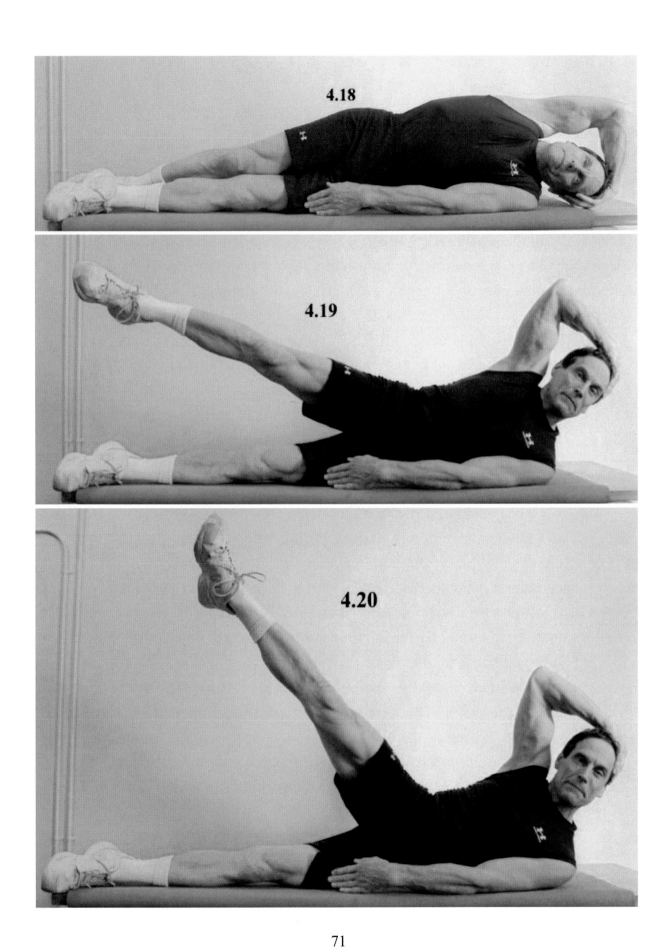

4.18

4.19

4.20

6. Pointer

a. Target Muscle Groups: Gluteus Maximus, Hamstrings, Erector Spinae

b. We have completed several exercises to develop strength and flexibility in the front and sides of our lower torso/hip complex. These muscle groups flex the human torso forward, bend it laterally, and turn it to either side. We have yet to address the muscles on the back side of the lower torso/hip complex, the muscles that extend our spine, shoulders, and hips. To execute gracefully and safely all the physical acts of daily life, we must strive always to develop balance and symmetry in our bodies. Fortunately, there is a simple exercise to challenge the muscles of the backside—Pointer.

c. Directions

(1) Position yourself on "all fours", your hands and knees shoulder-width apart and your head hanging down slightly (**Illustration 4.21**).

(2) As you begin to exhale, simultaneously:

i. raise your right arm in front of you and point straight ahead with your fingers;

ii. lift your head and look directly at where you are pointing;

iii. raise your left leg behind you, gradually straighten your knee, and point backward with the toes of your left foot. Pause momentarily in this position (**Illustration 4.22**).

(3) You should feel contractions in the muscles of your right upper back and rear shoulder, the back of your neck, your left lower back and left gluteus maximus, as well as a mild stretching in your left hamstring, the top of your left ankle, and your right latissimus dorsi.

(4) As you begin to inhale, return your right hand, head, left knee, and left foot to their respective beginning positions (**Illustration 4.21**). This completes one repetition on one side. Pause momentarily.

(5) Perform the same exercise using the opposite limbs. Lift your head as you point forward with your left hand and backward with your right foot (**Illustration 4.23**). Continue to alternate until you have completed 10 to 15 repetitions on each side.

(6) As you can feel, this exercise also helps us to develop better balance and agility, two important attributes of a truly healthy human being.

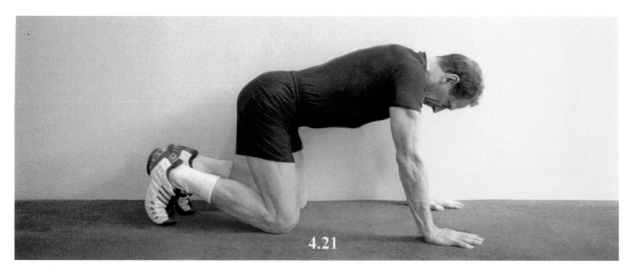

4.21

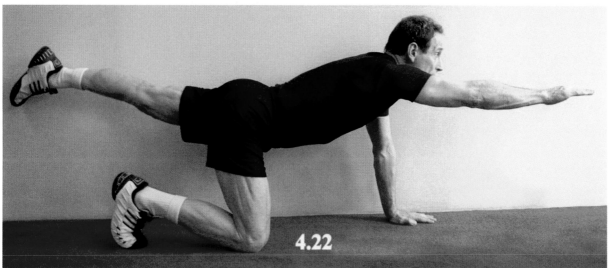

4.22

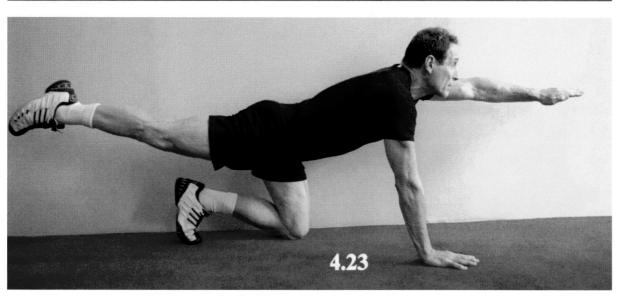

4.23

73

This completes the first level of training to develop a leaner and stronger lower torso/hip complex. This regimen should be performed a minimum of three days every week. It may be performed more often, even six days per week, if you so desire. Once you are able to eliminate exercises 2, 6, and 7— because they are included in exercises 4 and 8, respectively—you should be able to complete Abdominal Medley #1 in about 15 minutes. After a few weeks of regular performance, you will feel a significant difference, not just in how your clothes fit around your waistline, but also in how your body moves and responds as you go through the physical tasks of everyday life. You will feel better when you awaken in the morning and when you get in and out of a car. You will rake leaves and carry heavy grocery bags with more confidence and less fear. As your bodily awareness increases, you will begin to reclaim some of the energy you may have lost over the last few years or decades. You will begin to realize that you have the potential to be much stronger and much healthier for much longer in life than you had imagined previously. You are beginning to rediscover your strength for life.

Chapter 5

Abdominal Medley #2

Abdominal Medley #2

1. Agility Ball Lower Abdominal Curl and Leg Press

a. Primary Target Muscle Group: Lower Rectus Abdominis

b. Balancing on an agility ball and performing deep knee bends make this abdominal exercise more dynamic and challenging than the version on the floor. In addition to warming up your knee, ankle, hip, and lumbar joints, this exercise recruits several accessory muscle groups to maintain balance and develop better coordination.

c. Directions

(1) Sit on top of an agility ball with your knees bent and with your feet on the floor shoulder-width apart (**Illustration 5.1**).

(2) "Walk" forward in small steps as your buttocks descend toward the floor. Your knees will gradually bend to more than 100° as your gluteals come within a few inches of touching the floor. Allow your lower back to arch slightly against the lower front side of the ball. This is the beginning position (**Illustration 5.2**). Inhale.

(3) As you start to exhale, begin a lower abdominal curl, pushing your lower back forcefully into the ball while performing a leg press. **Illustration 5.3** is the halfway point.

(4) Keep pressing your lower back more and more firmly into the ball and continue the leg press until your knees are straight (**Illustration 5.4**). Pause momentarily in the "up" position.

(5) Inhale as you descend slowly back to the beginning position (**5.2**). Continue to press your lower back firmly into the ball.

(6) Repeat steps (3) to (5) for 10 to 20 repetitions. After the last repetition, remain in the topmost position (**Illustration 5.4**) in preparation for the next exercise in this medley.

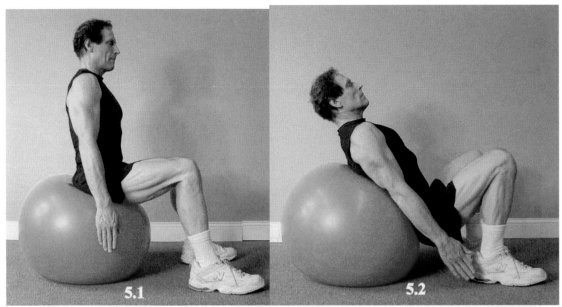

5.1　　5.2

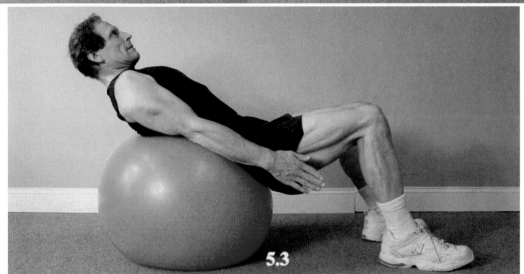

5.3

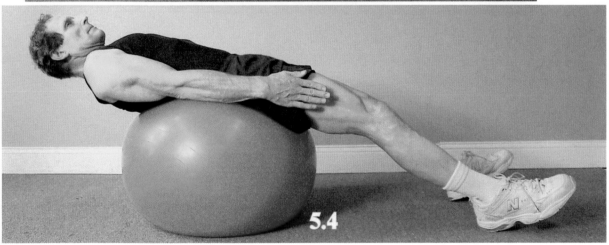

5.4

2. Agility Ball Upper Abdominal Curl

a. Primary Target Muscles: Upper and Lower Rectus Abdominis

b. As in the previous exercise, you will feel greater muscular challenge in exercising on an agility ball than on the floor. In particular, you will feel increasing tension in your upper rectus as you curl and then uncurl your head, neck, and shoulders at the beginning and end of this exercise.

c. Directions

(1) From the final position of the last exercise (**Illustration 5.4**), allow your lower spine to arch upward as you take a few small steps backward until your heels are approximately 12-18 inches from the ball. Your knees should be bent at approximately 90 degrees and your lower sternum over the center of the ball. Place the fingers of both hands behind your neck for support and allow your head to go backward and downward. **Illustration 5.5** is the beginning position. Keep your elbows back, in the same plane as your ears, and avoid pulling on your neck as you do this exercise. Inhale and pause.

(2) As you begin to exhale, first do a lower abdominal curl into the ball, then curl your head and chest forward and upward slowly and smoothly until your upper rectus muscles feel tightly contracted (**Illustration 5.6**). For most of us, this should be only about 10° to 30° above the horizontal plane of the floor, or until your shoulder blades just lose contact with the ball. Pause momentarily. At this stage of training do not try to go too high. Rise just to the point where your abdominals feel very strongly contracted.

(3) Begin to inhale as you uncurl your torso slowly to the beginning position, maintaining tension in your lower and upper recti all the way down to full extension of your neck and torso (**Illustration 5.5**). Pause momentarily.

(4) With precision and concentration, repeat steps (2) to (3) for 10-20 slow repetitions. Go directly into the next exercise because this is a medley; no need to rest when things are this exciting.

78

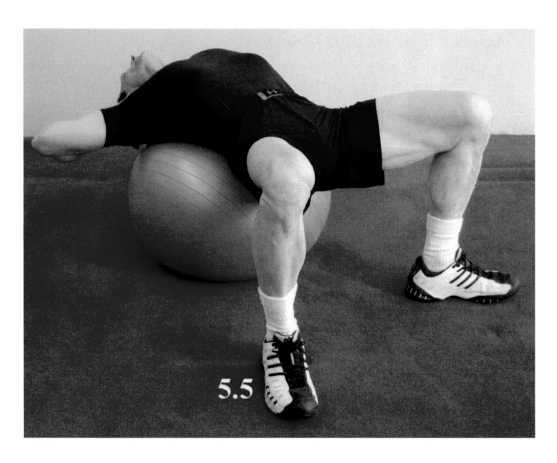

5.5

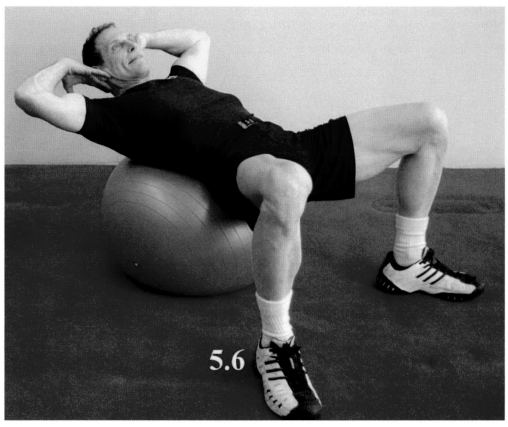

5.6

3. Agility Ball Alternating Diagonal Abdominal Curl

    a. Primary Target Muscles: External Obliques

    Secondary Target Muscles: Rectus Abdominis

    b. Because of the rotating motion of the torso in this exercise, we experience even greater excitement in our target and supporting muscles than we did in the previous exercise. By alternating side to side, we develop greater agility, a very important quality of life as we age.

    c. Directions

        (1) From the final position of the previous exercise (**Illustration 5.6**), leave your right hand behind your neck, turn your head to the right, look at your right elbow, and place your left hand next to your left hip. Allow your lower back to arch slightly and your right elbow to descend backward toward the floor. **Illustration 5.7** is the beginning position. Inhale deeply.

        (2) As you begin to exhale, first do a lower abdominal curl into the ball, then immediately curl your head, neck, right elbow and right shoulder upward and to the left, rotating toward the center of your body until your right elbow reaches a point approximately 18-24 inches above your naval or your symphysis pubis. **Illustration 5.8** is the peak position. Pause momentarily.

        (3) Inhale deeply as you uncurl your head, neck, right shoulder, and right elbow slowly toward but not to the beginning position. As you descend, place your left hand behind your neck so that both hands are supporting your head as you reach the centerline (**Illustration 5.9**).

        (4) Place your right hand next to your right hip and look to the left as your left elbow descends toward the floor (**Illustration 5.10**). Inhale.

        (5) Perform the exercise from left to right as you did from right to left.

        (6) Continue to alternate repetitions, turning your head to the right and curling up and to the left, then turning your head to the left and curling up and to the right. Do 10 to 15 repetitions to each side, then move directly to the next exercise of this exhilarating medley.

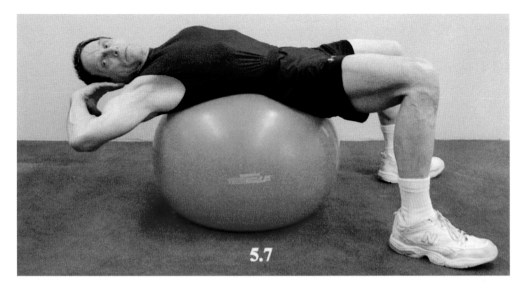

5.7

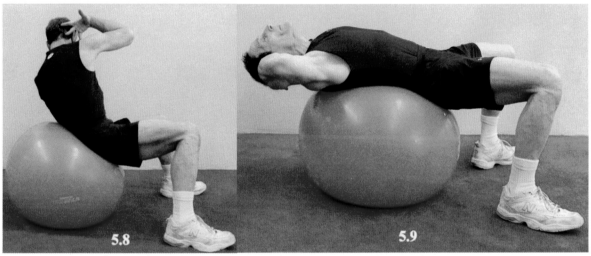

5.8

5.9

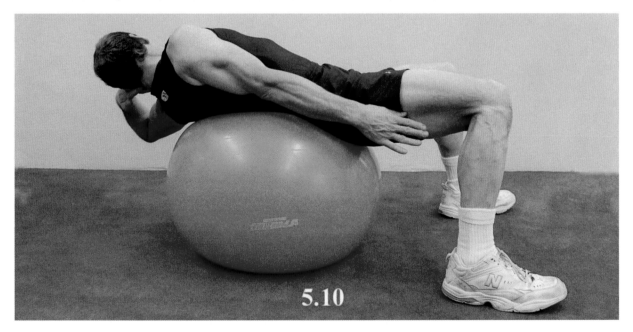

5.10

4. Abdominal Vacuums on Agility Ball.

a. Target Muscle: Transverse Abdominis.

b. We perform this exercise in a manner similar to the way in which we did it on the floor, except doing it on an agility ball requires more concentration.

c. Directions

(1) Recline on an agility ball with your hands at your sides (**Illustration 5.11**). Inhale as you allow your lower spine to arch upward and your abdomen to rise like bread dough (**Illustration 5.12**).

(2) Do not concern yourself at this time about the lower rectus down position. Our sole objective in this exercise is to engage the transverse abdominis as completely as possible. As you exhale, use your transverse abdominis to pull your lower and then your upper abdomen inward toward your spine and upward toward your sternum (**Illustration 5.13**). You should feel a hollowing of your entire abdominal cavity, from your pubic bone up to your lower rib cage.

(3) Hold this hollowed out position for 2 seconds.

(4) Repeat steps (1) to (3) for 10 repetitions in excellent form.

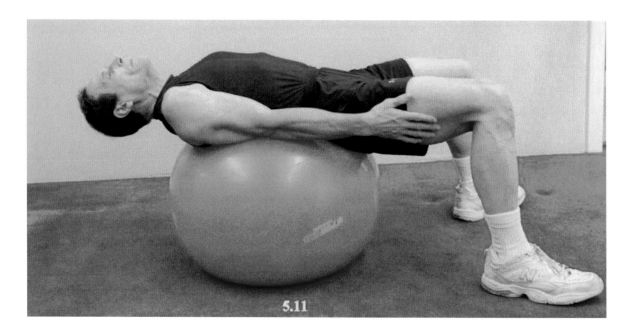

5.11

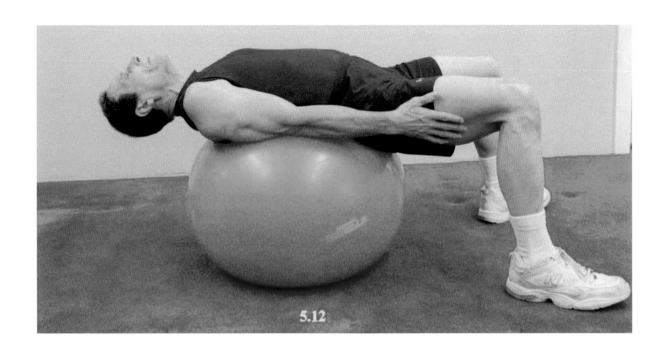

5.12

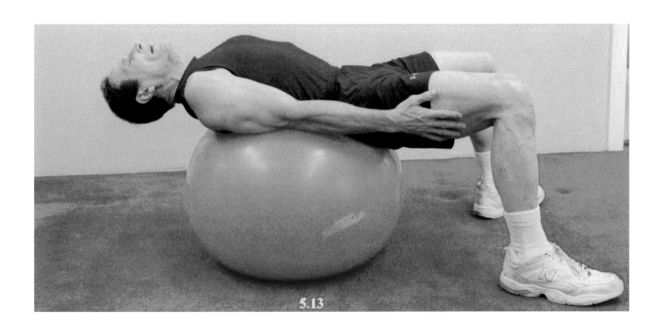

5.13

5. Side Jackknife on Agility Ball

a. Primary Target Muscles: Lateral External and Internal Obliques
Secondary Target Muscles: Gluteus Medius, Gluteus Minimus, and
Tensor Fascia Lata

b. This exercise helps us to develop even greater agility and coordination
than does the floor version.

c. Directions

(1) Lie on your left side over the top of the agility ball. Your left arm
is wrapped around the front edge of the ball. Your left hand is on the
floor and wedged under the front of the ball to prevent it from rolling.
Move your left foot forward about 12 inches, leaving your right leg in
line with your torso. The palm of your right hand should be on top of
your head and your fingertips should be touching the top of your left
ear. **Illustration 5.14** is the beginning position. Savor the feeling of a
great stretch along the entire right side of your body, especially from
your shoulder to your hip. Inhale.

(2) As you begin to exhale, lift your head, right shoulder, and right
elbow in an arcing motion upward and toward your right hip.
Simultaneously, do a side leg raise with your right leg, lifting your
right leg and foot laterally toward the ceiling. **Illustration 5.15** is
halfway.

(3) Pause momentarily in the peak position when your oblique and hip
abductor muscles feel strongly contracted (**Illustration 5.16**).

(4) As you begin to inhale, lower your right leg, head, and shoulders
back to their respective beginning positions (**Illustration 5.14**). Once
again enjoy the feeling of a fantastic stretch from your right shoulder
down to your right hip. All dynamic strength exercises are also
flexibility exercises—if we go slowly through a full range of motion
in each direction and pause briefly at each end of that range. After
pausing momentarily, perform steps (2)-(4) for 10 to 15 repetitions.
Repeat this exercise while lying on your right side.

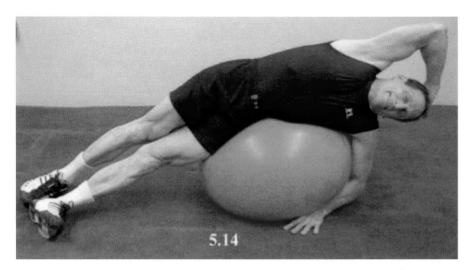

5.14

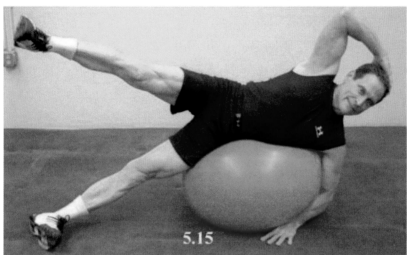

5.15

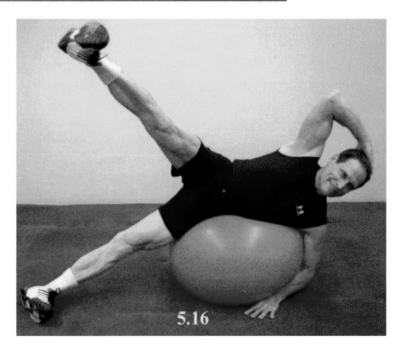

5.16

6. Agility Ball Pointer

a. Target Muscles: Erector Spinae, Gluteus Maximus, Hamstrings, Extensor muscles of the neck

b. Directions

(1) Lie face down on the ball such that your navel is over the center of the ball. Your arms hang straight down with your hands on the floor. Your knees are straight and your toes are touching the floor. Your head hangs down so that you are looking at the floor (**Illustration 5.18**). Inhale.

(2) As you begin to exhale, simultaneously lift your head, raise your right arm and shoulder, and extend your left leg and foot behind you. You should be pointing ahead with the fingers of your right hand and behind with the toes of your left foot. Your right arm and left leg are approximately parallel with the floor. Pause momentarily in the pointing position (**Illustration 5.19**).

(3) As you begin to inhale, lower your head, right hand, and left leg to their respective beginning positions (**Illustration 5.18**).

(4) Now perform the same exercise using the opposite extremities. As you begin to exhale, lift your head and simultaneously raise your left arm to point ahead and your right leg to point behind— until they are parallel with the floor (**Illustration 5.20**). Pause momentarily, then return again to the beginning position.

(5) Continue to alternate sides until you have performed 10 to 15 repetitions on each side.

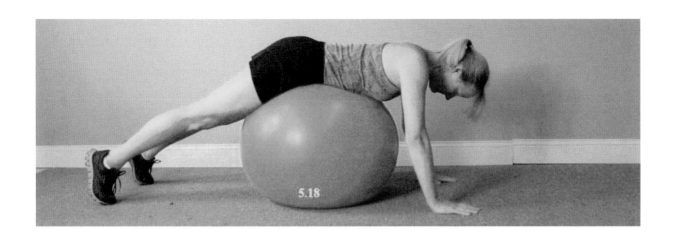

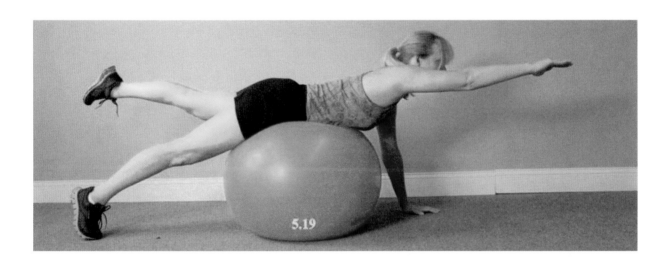

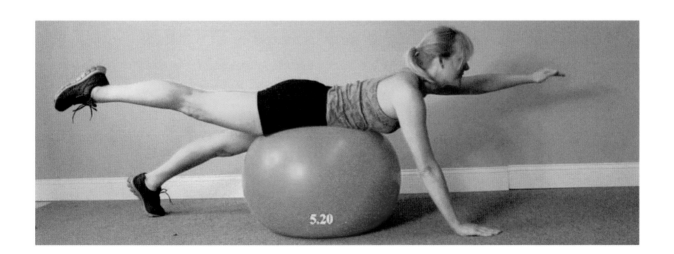

7. Reversely Rotating DNA Side Curl on Agility Ball

a. Primary Target Muscles: Transversospinalae, External and Internal Obliques; External Rotators of the Hip; Serratus Posterior
Secondary Target Muscles: Transverse Abdominis, Latissimus Dorsi, Posterior Deltoid, Quadratus Lumborum, Rotators of the Neck
b. Our goal here is to develop flexibility, power, and coordinated use in all the interrelated rotational muscles of the core.
c. Directions

(1) Lie on your left side on the ball, the tip of your lower sternum approximately over the center of the ball. Move your left foot 12 inches forward, your right foot 12 inches backward, and put your right hand behind neck. Lower and rotate your head, right shoulder, and elbow toward the floor as you turn your torso leftward and downward. Rotate your right hip internally so that your right big toe would be contacting the floor if you did not have a shoe on your foot. **Illustration 5.21** is the beginning position. Inhale.

(2) Begin to exhale as you lift your head, right shoulder, and elbow while turning your torso backward and upward. At the same time, externally rotate your right hip. **Illustration 5.22** is halfway up.

(3) Continue raising and rotating your head, right shoulder, elbow, hip, and torso upward and backward until your elbow points toward the ceiling (**Illustration 5.23**). Pause momentarily.

(4) Inhale as you allow all moving members of your body to return to their respective beginning positions (**Illustration 5.21**).

(5) Repeat Steps (2) – (4) for a total of 10 to 20 repetitions while lying on your left side, then perform an equal number of exciting repetitions while lying on your right side.

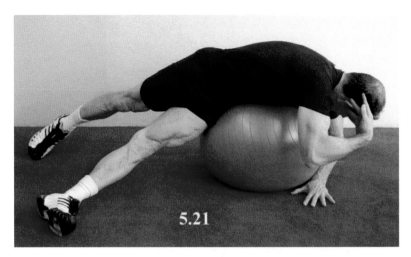

5.21

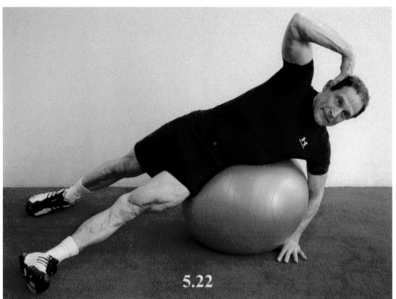

5.22

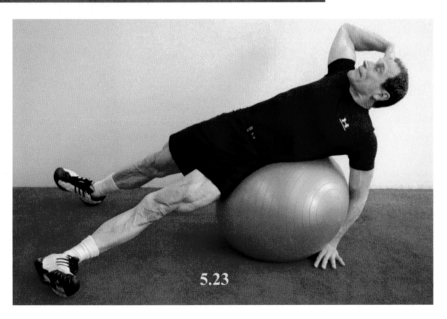

5.23

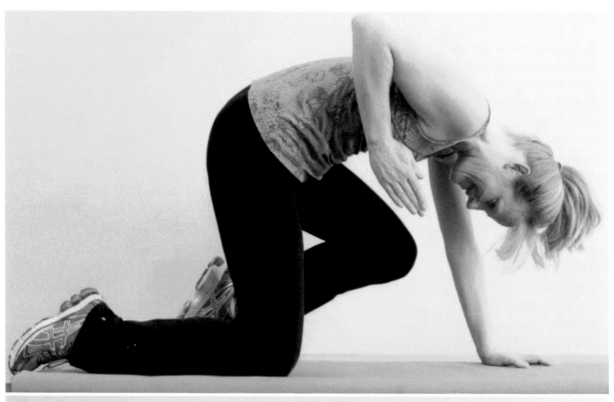

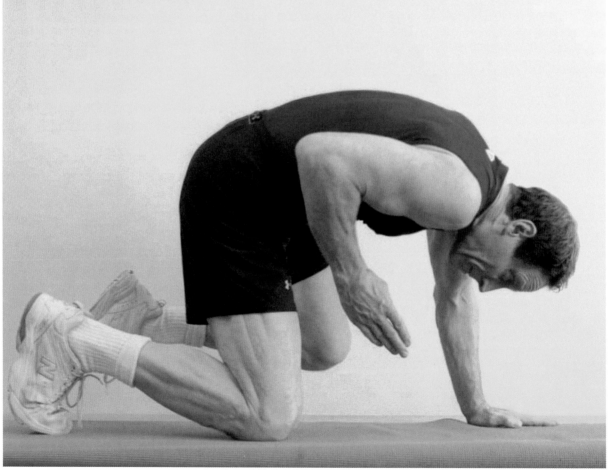

Chapter 6

Abdominal Medley #3

Abdominal Medley #3

1. Lower Ab Curl and Ab Vacuum with Knees Straight

    a. Target Muscles: Lower Rectus Abdominis and Transverse Abdominis

    b. By combining the Lower Abdominal Curl and the Abdominal Vacuum into a single exercise, we create a richer experience and save time as well. By performing this exercise with our legs straight, instead of with knees bent as in Medley #1, we approach abdominal nirvana.

    c. Directions

        (1) Lie on your back with your knees straight, arms at your sides, and your head against the floor. Inhale as you allow your abdominal muscles to relax and your spine to arch upward moderately. Pause momentarily (**Illustration 5.42**).

        (2) As you begin to exhale, use your transverse abdominis to pull your abdomen inward toward your spine (**Illustration 5.43**).

        (3) Continue to exhale as you perform a lower abdominal curl, pushing your lower back down firmly against the floor (**Illustration 5.44**). Pause momentarily in this position.

        (4) Inhale slowly as you return to the beginning position (**Illustration 5.42**). Pause momentarily, then repeat steps (2)-(4) until you have enjoyed 10-15 exciting repetitions. Proceed directly to the next exercise of this exhilarating medley.

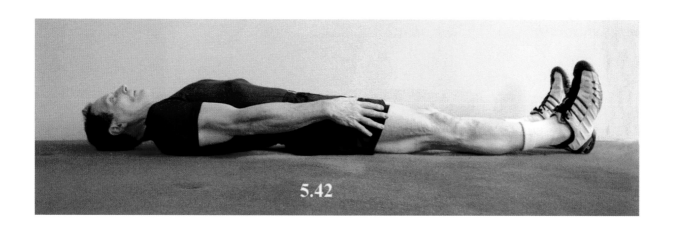

5.42

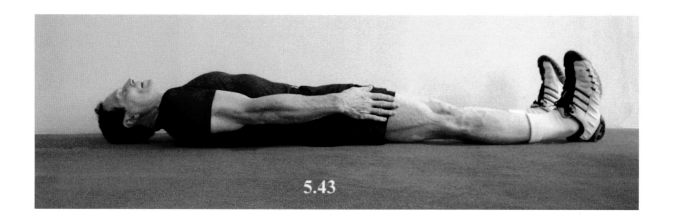

5.43

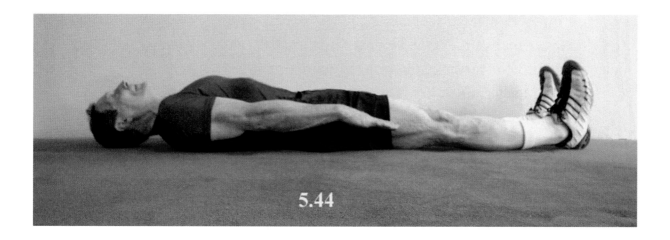

5.44

2. Upper Abdominal Curl and Vacuum, Knees Straight

a. Target Muscles: Upper and Lower Rectus Abdominis

Secondary Target Muscle Group: Transverse Abdominis

b. Here we intensify the upper abdominal curl by performing it with knees straight, by integrating the abdominal vacuum, and by maintaining the lower abdominal curl down position throughout the exercise.

c. Directions

(1) Lie on your back with your knees straight and your hands behind your head, your fingers supporting—but not pulling on—your neck. Perform a vacuum to pull your abdomen inward and upward. Follow immediately with a lower abdominal curl to push your lower back down firmly against the floor. **Illustration 5.45** is the beginning position. Inhale.

(2) As you begin to exhale, curl your head, shoulders, and chest upward and forward slowly until you feel your upper rectus abdominis contracted very tightly. You should feel your shoulder blades are just off the floor. Keep your elbows back to avoid pulling on your neck. Pause momentarily in the peak position, as though someone were about to punch you just above the navel **(Illustration 5.46)**. Keep your lower back pressed tightly to the floor throughout the entire exercise.

(3) As you begin to inhale, slowly uncurl your chest and shoulders toward their starting positions. As you do, use your transverse abdominis to pull your abdomen inward and upward until you reach the beginning position **(5.45)**.

(4) Pause momentarily in the down position. As you begin to exhale, repeat Steps (2) – (3) until you have completed 15-20 powerful repetitions. Proceed directly to the next exercise.

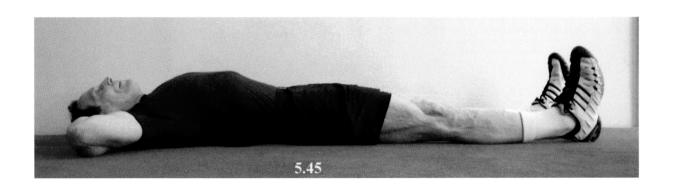

5.45

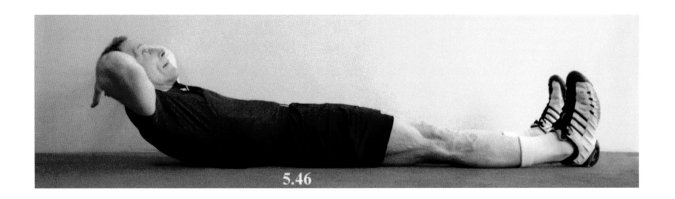

5.46

3. Diagonal Abdominal Curl with Vacuums and Hip Adduction

a. Primary Target Muscles: External Obliques, Upper and Lower Rectus Abdominis, Transverse Abdominis, Hip Adductors, Internal Obliques
b. In this version we change the positions and actions of the hips and integrate Abdominal Vacuums as we did in the previous exercise.
c. Directions

(1) Lie on the floor with knees bent, feet flat, right hand fingers reversed behind your neck, head to the right, and left hand on the floor next to your left hip. Do a pelvic tilt. Abduct your left hip until you feel a stretch in the groin on that side (**Illustration 5.47**). Inhale.

(2) As you exhale, curl your right shoulder, right elbow, and head upward, leftward, and toward the midline of your body. Feel for contractions in your right external obliques first, then in your right upper rectus as you prepare to be punched just above the navel. At the same time, maintain a powerful pelvic tilt and adduct your left hip so your left knee moves toward your navel (**Illustration 5.48).**

(3) Continue to curl your right elbow as far as you can to the left and to move your left knee as far as you can to the right. Both may cross the midline of your body. **Illustration 5.49** is the fully contracted position. Pause for two seconds.

(4) As you begin to inhale, slowly uncurl all moving members of your body back to their respective beginning positions. As you do, use your transverse abdominis to perform a vacuum, pulling your abdomen inward and upward during your descent (**Illustration 5.47**). In this exercise, we challenge the upper and lower rectus, transverse abdominis, obliques, and left hip adductors simultaneously.

(5) When you reach the beginning position, you should feel a great stretch in all of your target muscle groups, including the adductor muscles of your left inner thigh.

(6) Pause momentarily in this stretched position and then perform up to 20 repetitions on this side by repeating Steps (2)-(5).

(7) Repeat this exercise on the opposite side.

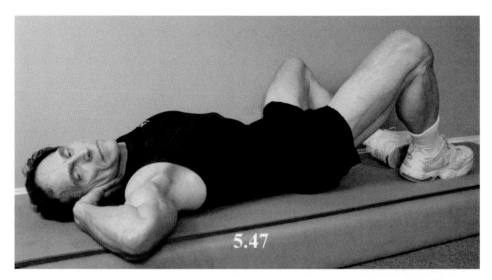

5.47

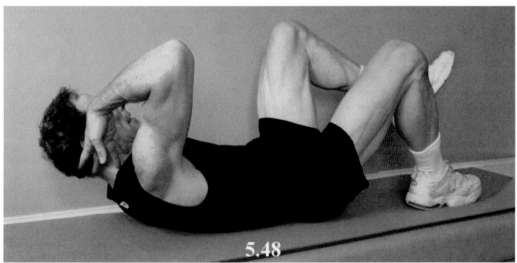

5.48

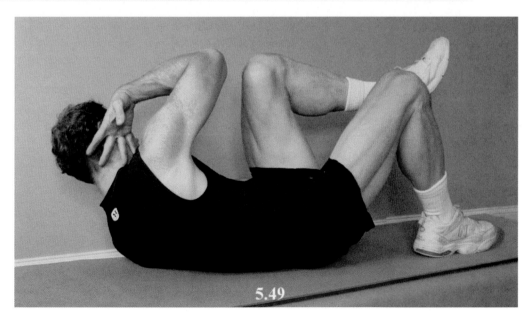

5.49

97

4. DNA Rotating Side Curl with Vacuums

a. Primary Target Muscles: External Obliques
Secondary Muscles: Upper Rectus and Transverse Abdominis
b. This exercise isolates the external oblique muscles in their primary vector of contraction, which is downward and medial from the lateral lower rib cage toward the midline of the abdomen.
c. Directions

(1) Lie on your left side with the fingers of your right hand reversed behind your neck. Your left hand rests just in front of your left hip.

(2) The medial aspects of your knees are touching each other, but your right lower leg and foot are extended 12 inches ahead and your left lower leg and foot are positioned 12 inches rearward, causing your legs to cross in an "X".

(3) Turn your head, right arm, and shoulder to the right, backward, and downward toward the floor behind you, until your torso is rotated as far to that side as is comfortable. Using transverse abdominis, execute an abdominal vacuum. This is the beginning position (**Illustration 5.50**). Your body is spiraled in a manner vaguely suggestive of DNA. You should feel a great stretch in your right external obliques.

(4) As you begin to exhale, rotate your head, right shoulder, and right elbow forward, upward, and to the left, toward the midline of your body. **Illustration 5.51** is the halfway point. You should feel strong contractions in your right external obliques.

(5) Continue to rotate your torso upward and to the left until your right elbow is pointed directly to the ceiling (**Illustration 5.52**). Pause momentarily in this position.

(6) As you begin to inhale, lower your right shoulder slowly back to the beginning position. At the same time, use your transverse abdominis to pull your abdomen inward again (**Illustration 5.50**).

(7) When you reach the beginning position, pause momentarily, then begin to exhale and repeat steps (4) through (6). Do up to 20 repetitions while on your left side and then do the same on your right.

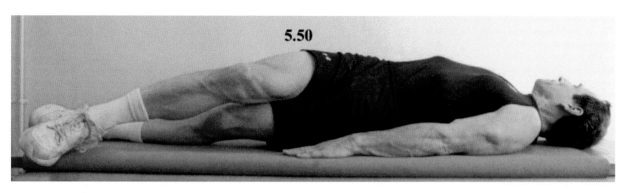

5.50

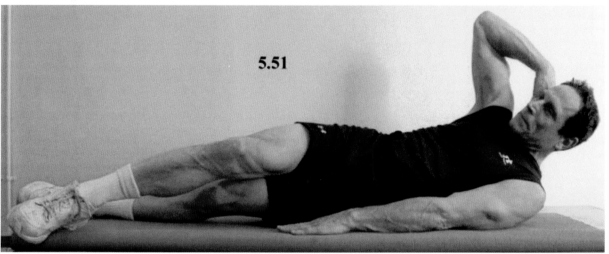

5.51

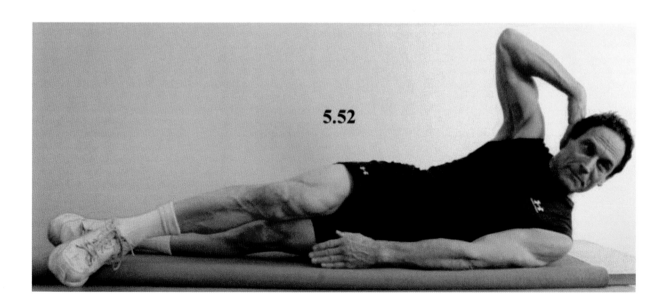

5.52

5. Pointer Head to Toe

a. Primary Target Muscle Groups: Extensor muscles of the spine and hips.
b. This is an advanced version of the simple pointer in Ab Medley #1. It provides dynamic stimulation of the muscles from the back of your neck to the bottom of your toes.
c. Directions

(**1**) Begin in the all-fours position—on your hands and knees and looking down at the floor. Your toes should be dorsiflexed so that you feel a stretch of the muscles on the bottom of your feet and toes and in your Achilles tendons. This is the beginning position (**Illustration 5.54**).

(**2**) As you begin to inhale, bring your right elbow backward, your left knee forward, and your chin toward your chest (**Illustration 5.55**). You should feel a great stretch from the back of your head to the bottom of your spine. Pause momentarily.

(**3**) As you begin to exhale, simultaneously: raise your head to look straight ahead; raise your right arm, straighten your elbow, and point at a spot directly ahead; and extend your left leg straight backward, pointing your toes backward as far as you can (**Illustration 5.56**). Pause momentarily.

(**4**) Return to the beginning position.

(**5**) As you begin to inhale, repeat steps (2) through (4) on the opposite side, that is: first bring your left elbow backward; bend your right knee as you bring it forward; and flex your head toward your abdomen. After pausing momentarily in this flexed position, begin to exhale as you: extend your left arm to point straight ahead; extend your right leg to point straight behind; and lift your head to look ahead.

(**6**) Continue to alternate sides until you have completed 10 to 15 repetitions on each side.

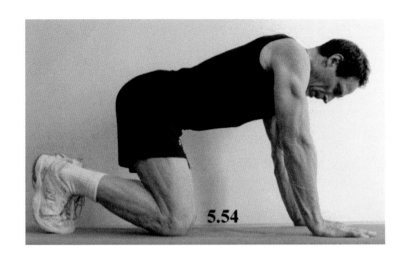

5.54

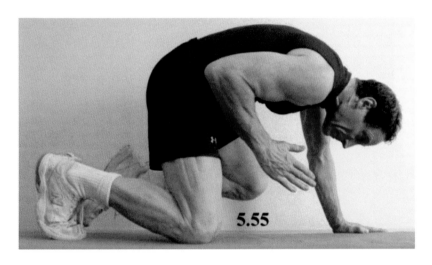

5.55

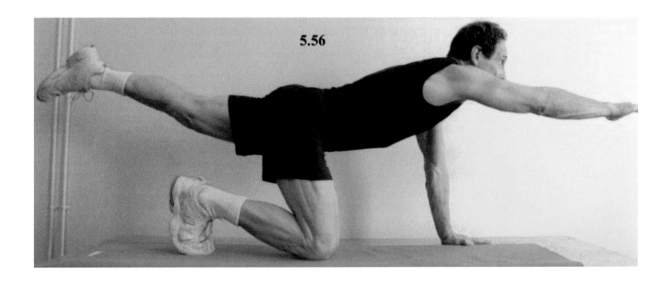

5.56

101

6. Backup

a. Primary Target Muscle Group: Lower Erector Spinae
Secondary Target Groups: Quadratus Lumborum, Gluteus Maximus
b. If you are going to develop great strength in your abdominals, the flexors of the spine, it is common sense that you should also develop strength in the extensors of the spine. Achieving a balance in these opposing muscle groups is one of the keys to attaining and maintaining good posture. Great posture not only helps to make your abdomen appear leaner, it also plays a critical role in your long-term health. If you have a history of lower spinal injuries or pain, you should consult a knowledgeable training advisor and/or doctor before attempting this exercise.
c. Directions

(1) Lie face down across a padded table or bench so that your buttocks, hips, and thighs are just off one side. Stabilize your torso and upper body by holding onto the other side of the bench.
(2) Your knees point to the floor and are bent at 90° so that your lower legs point backward, approximately parallel with the floor (**Illustration 5.58**). Inhale.
(3) As you begin to exhale, raise your legs and buttocks slowly upward, so that your thighs approach—but do not exceed—the plane of your torso. Keep your knees bent at 90°. You should feel a tightening (but not pain) in the muscles of your lower back and gluteals (**Illustration 5.59**). Pause momentarily.
(4) As you inhale, slowly lower your legs back to the beginning position. You should feel a mild traction-like stretch in the erector spinae muscles of your lower back.
(5) Do 5 to 10 slow repetitions of this exercise. If you have any lower back pain or discomfort during or after the performance of this exercise, leave it out of your training at this time.

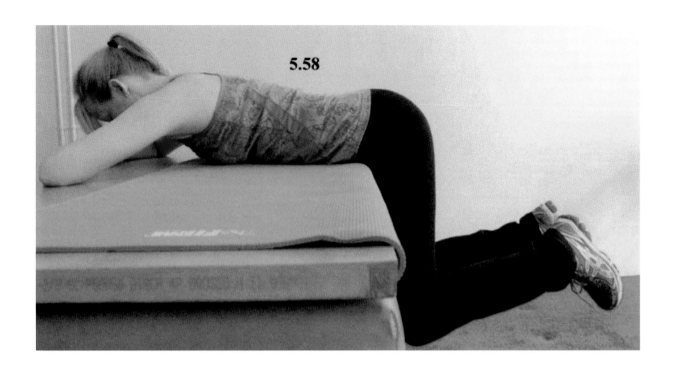

5.58

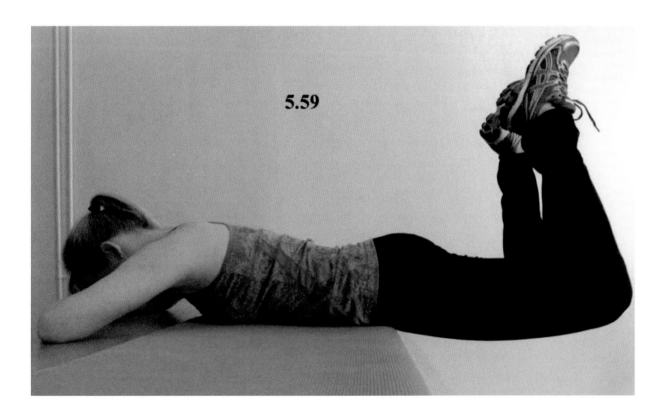

5.59

7. DNA Side Jackknife with External Hip Rotation

a. Target Muscle Groups: External Obliques; Gluteus Medius and Minimus, Tensor Fascia Lata

b. In this exercise we combine two previous exercises, the DNA Side Curl and the Side Jackknife, and add external rotation of the hip to create an even higher level of exercise excitement.

c. Directions

(1) Lie on your left side with your knees straight, your right foot in front of your left, and the right hip and ankle rotated inwardly so that only the big toe area of your right shoe contacts the floor. With your right hand behind your neck, turn your right shoulder backward and downward so that your right elbow moves close to the floor **Illustration 5.60** is the beginning position. Inhale.

(2) Begin to exhale and, simultaneously, raise your right ankle and turn your right shoulder forward and toward the ceiling. As you raise your right leg and ankle, gradually rotate your right foot outward, so that your big toe is turning upward. **Illustration 5.61** is halfway up.

(3) Continue exhaling as you raise your right shoulder and right ankle closer to the ceiling, all the while turning your right foot outward. When you feel tight contractions in the muscles on the right side of your torso and on the side and back of your right hip, you have reached peak contraction. Your big toe should be pointed almost directly to the ceiling (**Illustration 5.62**). Pause momentarily.

(4) As you begin to inhale, retrace your upward movements. Uncurl your shoulder and lower your leg as you rotate your right big toe inwardly back slowly to the beginning positions.

(5) Enjoy 10 to 15 focused repetitions while lying on your left side, then repeat the feat with equal focus while lying on your right side.

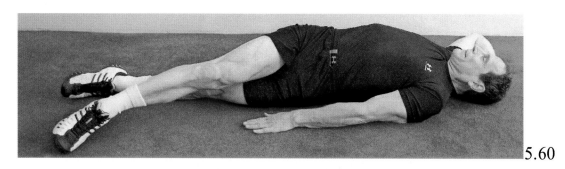

5.60

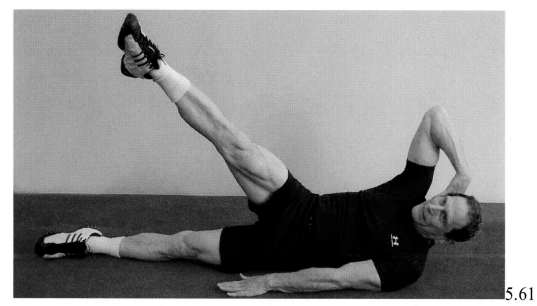

5.61

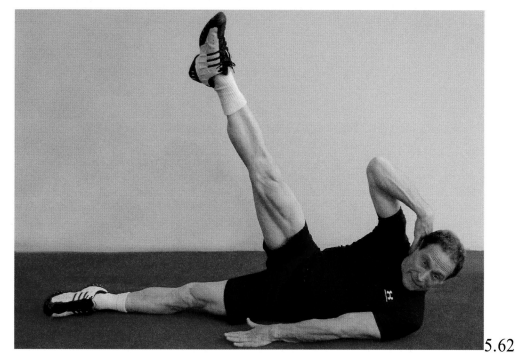

5.62

Your Weekly Core Muscle Strengthening Plan

You are now the proud lessee of three distinct, but highly related, core muscle routines. You are on your way to stardom in the development of stronger muscles throughout your entire lower torso/hip complex, especially your abdominals.

However, you do not own these workouts outright; you are only leasing them. You may use them for as long in your life as you are willing to pay your weekly "rent;" that is, for as long as you perform these exercises regularly every week. The next question might be:

How often should you do these exercises?

Please consider the following recommendations for your core workouts.

1. Do only one of these workouts on any given day. What matters most is that you do a few exercises well, as opposed to trying to do as many as possible. More is not better. Better is better. Therefore, make the most of the exercises in one workout and limit yourself to the target range of repetitions recommended.

2. Do all three of these core muscle workouts on a rotating basis. Do not abandon Abdominal Medley #1 just because you can now do #2 and #3. By continuing to do the first workout once or twice weekly, you stay grounded in the basics. If you do this, you will discover increasing benefits from these basic exercises.

3. Perform each of these three workouts at least once per week. If you have the time in your busy life, do each medley twice per week. However, always give yourself one day off from core training each week. That way, if you miss a day because of some unforeseen interruption, you have no reason to feel guilty; it was just your day off that week. In addition, when you take one day off from core training each week, you will appreciate just how great they feel on the days when you do perform them.

Part III

Leaner for Life

Chapter 7   *The American Diet Revolution!*

Chapter 8.   *Cardiorespiratory Conditioning*

Chapter 9   *Whole-Body Strength for Life®*
                Training

Introduction to Part III

As effective as core muscle exercises can be for building strength, they are not by themselves effective for reducing the circumference of your midsection. To make your waist smaller and your entire body leaner, you must do more than core exercises. By far, the most significant factors in becoming leaner are the (1) types of foods you eat and (2) whether those foods stimulate your body to pack more fat into your fat cells or, instead, they signal your body to release and burn some of the fat already stored in those cells. Chapter 7 provides dietary guidance enabling you to become an engine that burns fat rather than a warehouse that stores oodles of it.

Although your diet is pre-eminent, you can augment your quest to be leaner by engaging in two other exciting exercise experiences, cardiorespiratory conditioning and whole-body strength training. Chapters 8 and 9, respectively, outline the principles for success in these two fabulous physical pursuits.

As mentioned previously, each of these three disciplines is worthy of and demands full treatment in an entire book, far beyond the space available in the present volume. For this reason, Chapters 7 through 9 provide only brief descriptions of these subjects. However, I hope these summaries inspire you to study each of these disciplines in greater depth in the very near future.

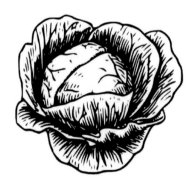

Chapter 7

The American Diet Revolution!

In the previous six chapters, you learned how you can develop more powerful core muscles as you age, even if you are 50, 60, 70, 80, or in your 90s. However, you learned also that you will not attain middle-of-the body leanness if your only strategy to reach this goal is doing core muscle exercises. The most important tactic to being leaner is to avoid eating foods that cause you to store body fat. Based upon the recommendations of honest nutritional researchers of the 21st Century, this chapter is a clear-cut guide to the types of foods you must avoid if your goal is to reduce your current level of body fat. Just as importantly, in this guide you will also discover a rich array of nutritious foods which enhance your health as you add them to your diet.

Many Americans claim they "eat well." If this were true, 2/3 of our adult population would not be obese or pathologically overweight. A majority of us eat foods that stimulate the accumulation of body fat, especially around our abdomens. In short, we have serious, complex, and wide-spread dietary problems. Although going "low-carb" or "Paleo" can be very helpful for some people, for most of us, these approaches are not enough. If we are to succeed in returning to levels of relative leanness of American adults in the 1950s, a full-blooded revolution in our diets is required. This must be a revolution not only about the foods we eat, but also, in what we think about the foods we eat.

Three years ago, as I began writing *Abdominal Strength for Life®!*, I planned to include a brief dietary advice chapter of about 20 pages to guide readers toward reducing, rather than accumulating, body fat. However, after months of research, it was clear that the 20-page "chapter" would have to be about 200 pages in length. Therefore, I suspended work on the present book while I composed an in-depth study of nutritional advice, weight loss, and dietary recommendations in the United States. The result of this effort is *American Diet Revolution! (ADR!),* published by Morgan James and scheduled for first release on February 12, 2019. If you really want to understand why and how the Standard American Diet (SAD) of the 20th Century caused obesity and diabetes rates in the US to rise to their current levels, you will find answers in this book.

In the meantime, until you are ready to study *ADR!,* in the next few pages you will encounter "The Pro-Active, Two-Page, Strength for Life®, Every-Single-Day, Eating-for-Well-Being Guide." In a clear and compact format, this guide enumerates specific foods you should eat and specific foods you should avoid in order to reach your personal goals for leanness and good health. This is followed by a very useful instrument to monitor your dietary progress: "The Strength for Life® One-Week Nutritional Diary." By documenting for yourself everything you eat for seven days, you will be able to judge how well you are following the recommendations in the guide.

For several years in my clinic, the Strength for Life® Health and Fitness Center, I have used this two-page guide and the nutritional diary to help thousands of patients and exercise trainees succeed in reducing their body fat to healthful levels. You too can achieve leaner and stronger abdominals by using these tools conscientiously.

One word of caution regarding use of the Eating-for-Well-Being Guide: you should not feel obligated to follow every dietary recommendation immediately. The guide is divided into three sections. Section A is a list of several of highly nutritious foods you should attempt to introduce gradually into your diet. From this section, each week select one food that you are not eating currently and give it a try. If you like it, add it to your repertoire of favorite healthy foods. If not, move on. The following week, try another new food from Section A.

Conversely, Section C is a detailed list of foods that will cause you to gain fat weight and, therefore, should be eliminated from your diet. From this section, each week select one food that you consume at present and ban it forever.

What's in Section B? It lists foods that are nutritious and delicious, but which should be consumed in limited quantities or only occasionally. The foods you add to your diet from Sections A and B will replace the toxic foodstuffs in Section C that you will be slowly eliminating from your life.

The Pro-Active, Two-Page, Strength for Life®, Every-Single-Day, Eating-for-Well-Being Guide

A. <u>What</u> <u>We</u> <u>Must</u> <u>Eat</u> and <u>Drink</u>: the Essentials

1. Eat 7-10 servings of fresh, organic vegetables, including

    a. a large salad with raw, leafy green, and brightly colored vegetables;

    b. at least one full cup of lightly cooked vegetables and/or soup;

    c. at least two ounces of fermented vegetables, such as sauerkraut.

2. Eat several servings of organic and/or pastured-raised fats, including:

    a. at least two tablespoons each of coconut and olive oils; and

    b. at least 2-4 ounces of raw seeds, nuts, and/or avocado; or

    c. 2-3 ounces of animal fat from eggs/meat or fish (ova/omnivores)

3. Eat 2-4 small-to-moderate portions of organic/pasture-raised proteins:

    a. two to three eggs, if you are an ova-lactivore or omnivore;

    b. several servings of raw nuts and seeds, more if you are a vegan;

    c. one serving of bone, meat, or fish protein, if you are an omnivore.

4. Drink at least three pints of pure water—one pint between all meals.

5. Drink at least two servings nutritional beverages, such as:

    a. 1-2 cups of bone broth, if you are an omnivore; or

    b. 1-2 cups of a high-mineral vegetable broth or drink;

    c. 8-16 ounces of a nutritional smoothie, especially post-exercise;

    d. home-made, vegetable-rich, and/or bone-broth-based soups.

B. <u>What</u> <u>We</u> <u>May</u> <u>Eat</u> <u>or</u> <u>Drink:</u> the Optionals

1. 1-2 servings of a low-sugar fruit, such as, berries or ½ of a small apple;

2. 1-2 cups of coffee, tea, or kombucha, and 3-6 ounces of organic red wine;

3. 1-4 ounces of pasture-raised butter, cheese, sour cream, whole-milk yogurt;

4. 1-2 ounces of an organic chocolate bar, at least 80% cacao and low-sugar;

5. 2-3 ounces of cooked quinoa, fermented organic soy, or baked sweet potato,

6. and, once per week, a "goof" (e.g., ice cream at your favorite parlor).

C. <u>What</u> <u>We</u> <u>Must</u> <u>Eliminate:</u> the Toxins

1. All processed, non-organic, synthetically sweetened, flavored, colored, and preserved, or genetically modified foods, including but not limited to:
   a. any industrial foodstuffs derived from plants treated with herbicides, pesticides, fungicides, or chemical fertilizers; and
   b. any foods from animals treated with antibiotics or growth stimulants, or fed chemically raised grains or other toxins;

2. All grain-based foodstuffs, including: breads, pasta, cereals, oatmeal, bagels, granola, crackers, cookies, pizza, muffins, scones, pies, cakes;

3. All sugar-intense or artificially sweetened: beverages—such as, fruit juices, soda, and sweetened teas, coffees, or sports drinks; or solid foods—such as: candies, cookies, pastries, low-fat and non-fat dairy products, or foodstuffs sweetened with high-fructose corn syrup and facsimiles;

4. All high-starch pseudo-vegetable foods, such as: corn, potatoes, chips, most beans, French fries, popcorn, and other industrial snack "foods".

5. All foods containing industrial, high Omega-6, pseudo-vegetable oils, such as: corn, soybean, cottonseed, canola, safflower, peanut, sunflower, etc.

6. As much as possible, any foods or drinks that cause GI distress, such as gas or bloating, or are sold in metal cans, plastic bags, or plastic containers.

Strength for Life® One-week Nutritional Diary

Name _____   Dates: ___/___ to ___/___/___

Day One: ___/___   **Day Two:** ___/___

Pre-breakfast: Water, _____   **Pre-Breakfast:** Water, _____

       Breakfast   time: ___   **Breakfast**   time: ___

Vegetables: _____   Vegetables: _____

Fats: _____   Fats: _____

Protein: _____   Protein: _____
Other: _____   Other: _____

       Snack: **Snack:**

Water, _____   Water, _____

       Lunch   time:_____   **Lunch**   time: ____

Vegetables: _____   Vegetables: _____

Fats: _____   Fats: _____

Protein: _____   Protein: _____
Other: _____   Other: _____

       Snack: **Snack:**

Water, _____   Water, _____

       Dinner   time: _____   **Dinner**   time: ____

Vegetables: _____   Vegetables: _____

Fats: _____   Fats: _____

Protein: _____   Protein: _____
Other: _____   Other: _____

Post-dinner: _____   **Post-dinner:** _____

Day Three: __/_

Pre-Breakfast: Water, _____

       Breakfast   time: ___

Vegetables: _____

Fats: _____

Protein: _____

Other: _____

       Snack:

Water, _____

       Lunch   time: ____

Vegetables: _____

Fats: _____

Protein: _____

Other: _____

       Snack:

Water, _____

       Dinner   time: ____

Vegetables: _____

Fats: _____

Protein: _____

Other: _____

Post-dinner: _____

Day Four: __/_

Pre-Breakfast: Water, _____

       Breakfast   time: ___

Vegetables: _____

Fats: _____

Protein: _____

Other: _____

       Snack:

Water, _____

       Lunch   time: ____

Vegetables: _____

Fats: _____

Protein: _____

Other: _____

       Snack:

Water, _____

       Dinner   time: ____

Vegetables: _____

Fats: _____

Protein: _____

Other: _____

Post-dinner: _____

Day Five: __/_

Pre-Breakfast: Water, _____

Breakfast   time: ___

Vegetables: _____

Fats: _____

Protein: _____

Other: _____

Snack:

Water, _____

Lunch   time: _____

Vegetables: _____

Fats: _____

Protein: _____

Other: _____

Snack:

Water, _____

Dinner   time: _____

Vegetables: _____

Fats: _____

Protein: _____

Other: _____

Post-dinner: _____

Day Six: __/_

Pre-Breakfast: Water, _____

Breakfast   time: ___

Vegetables: _____

Fats: _____

Protein: _____

Other: _____

Snack:

Water, _____

Lunch   time: _____

Vegetables: _____

Fats: _____

Protein: _____

Other: _____

Snack:

Water, _____

Dinner   time: _____

Vegetables: _____

Fats: _____

Protein: _____

Other: _____

Post-dinner: _____

Day Seven: __/_

Pre-Breakfast: Water, _____

Breakfast   time: ___

Vegetables: _____

Fats: _____

Protein: _____

Other: _____

Snack:

Water, _____

Lunch   time: ____

Vegetables: _____

Fats: _____

Protein: _____

Other: _____

Snack:

Water, _____

Dinner   time: ____

Vegetables: _____

Fats: _____

Protein: _____

Other: _____

Post-dinner: _____

Overview of Current Weekly Diet

Strengths

Raw veg? Fermented? Cooked?

Clean proteins? Good Fats?

_____

_____

_____

Weaknesses

Processed "foods"?
Grain-based foodstuffs? (Bread, bagels, chips, muffins, oatmeal, corn bread, cereals, sodas, cookies, crackers, and other processed grass-seed products?
High sugar dairy products?
Sugary liquids (sodas, fruit juices)?

_____

_____

_____

Self-recommended Dietary Changes

_____

_____

_____
__

Chapter 8

Cardiorespiratory Conditioning

Many of us who are American adults believe performing long bouts of "cardio" exercise is the most important thing we can do to shed excess body fat. A sizeable percentage of us in this group believe further that doing "cardio" exercise exclusively is all we need to do to become leaner. Unfortunately, over the past few decades, most up-to-date physiologists, researchers, and exercise advisors have shown conclusively that doing only "cardio" is not a successful strategy to become lean.

From a statistical perspective, as science writer Gary Taubes has documented, when we burn more calories through exercise, we consume more calories from food. Therefore, merely burning more calories—by exercising more intensively or for longer durations—is not necessarily a reliable measure of how well we will reduce excess body fat. As cardiologist and author Dr. William Davis has observed and described, a surprisingly high percentage of amateur triathletes—most of whom do "cardio" exercise many hours every week—are overweight. In short, most of us will not become significantly leaner, if our approach to this goal is predominantly or exclusively doing "cardio" exercise.

Although doing "cardio" is not by itself an efficient tool for decreasing excess body fat, doing exercises that stimulate your cardiovascular and respiratory systems simultaneously does enhance your health in many other significant ways. It can lower your blood pressure levels, improve circulation in your arteries and veins, stimulate digestive movements in your colon, improve the flow of air through your respiratory passages, decrease feelings of anxiety or depression, stimulate creative thinking, and increase the strength and flexibility of smooth and cardiac muscle throughout your entire cardiorespiratory system. In other words, even if it is not the ultimate way to burn stored body fat, cardiorespiratory exercise, when performed regularly and intelligently, improves your health significantly.

What is the cardiorespiratory system? Anatomically, rather than one system, your cardiorespiratory system is where and how two distinct systems of your body meet, overlap, and interact to deliver oxygen to every cell you own.

The cardiovascular system is comprised mainly of your heart, which is primarily cardiac muscle, and your blood vessels, the walls of which contain smooth muscular coats. The pre-eminent job of cardiac muscle is to generate the force necessary to initiate blood flow through the arterial circuitry of your body. Blood flow makes possible the delivery of nutrients—especially oxygen—to your ever-hungry cells. Contractions by smooth muscles in your arteries assist in blood flow. Once oxygen and other nutrients have been delivered, your cardiovascular system must return depleted blood back to your heart. Unlike your arteries, the smooth muscle coats in your veins are thin and relatively weak. Alternating contraction and relaxation by your diaphragm and by the muscles of your legs and core generate the forces necessary to complete the return voyage of depleted blood to your heart. It is not coincidental that most "cardio" exercises require repeated strenuous contractions by the diaphragm and by the muscles of your lower extremities and thorax.

The respiratory system is composed of passageways through which air comes in through your mouth and nose, makes its way down and into your lungs, gives up its oxygen in exchange for carbon dioxide, then flows upward and exits via the same passageways through which in entered only moments before. The muscular force for inspiration is generated primarily by the underlying diaphragm. As this internal skeletal muscle contracts, it moves downward, creating a partial vacuum in the thoracic cavity which triggers inspiration. During strenuous exercise, as you attempt to inspire more air than when you are sedentary, your diaphragm contracts more forcefully and moves downward farther than it does normally. Challenging your respiratory system in this manner regularly increases the amount of air you can take into your lungs with each inhalation. When inspiration is complete, the diaphragm relaxes, moves upward, and, with assistance of the intercostal and abdominal muscles, allows you to exhale as forcefully as you inspired a few seconds before.

The cardiorespiratory system is the highly coordinated manner in which the cardiovascular and respiratory systems meet and exchange gases in the alveolar sacs of the lungs. This is certainly one of the most important biological events in human life. One could argue this function, which is improved significantly by consistent cardiorespiratory exercise, is far more important than decreasing excessive stores of body fat. Therefore, let's review cardiorespiratory function in slightly more detail.

The first phase of cardiorespiratory circulation occurs when you inhale air through your nose and mouth from the environment around you. That air then makes its way to your lungs, where oxygen is extracted in the alveolar sacs and transferred to very small blood vessels, the capillaries. Oxygen-enriched blood flows to your heart, where powerful cardiac muscle contractions pump the nutrient-rich blood out through your arteries to every cell in your body. As your cells take up and use oxygen and other nutrients to fulfill their metabolic functions, they discharge waste products, especially carbon dioxide.

In the second phase of cardiorespiratory circulation, small veins pick up carbon dioxide and other metabolic wastes of cell metabolism and transport them to larger and then even larger veins. With assistance from muscle contractions in your core, intercostal, and leg muscles, and from pressure gradients created by movements of your diaphragm, depleted venous blood returns to your heart. This oxygen-poor blood is then pumped to your lungs. By gaseous exchange in the alveolar sacs, carbon dioxide waste is downloaded and incoming oxygen is uploaded. As you exhale, offloaded carbon dioxide and other wastes are discharged into the environment and the cardiorespiratory cycle is complete.

When you exercise to improve your cardiorespiratory circulation, you are striving for cardiorespiratory fitness. How can you do this?

Five Ways to Improve Your Cardiorespiratory Fitness

1. Practice deep breathing. Every time you exert yourself physically, inhale slowly and deeply through your nose and exhale slowly and completely through your mouth. Inhaling and exhaling in this slightly exaggerated manner promotes powerful contraction and relaxation of the diaphragm and of the skeletal muscles between your ribs (intercostals). Consistent deep breathing during strenuous physical activities improves your ability to take in more air, and hence more oxygen, per inhalation. Soon will you develop the habit of breathing in and out easily and deeply, even when you are sedentary or mildly active. No longer will you need to "catch your breath" after climbing a couple flights of stairs.

2. Every single day, try to do at least 20 minutes of continuous, low-level, physical exercise. What is low-level exercise? Good examples are: taking a

brisk walk, riding your bike, or working in your yardall at a pace you can sustain easily for the entire 20 minutes without stopping to rest. Of course, if you want to exert yourself for longer than 20 minutes, do so; but remind yourself always that the first 20 minutes are the most important. You cannot go for 40 minutes, unless first you go for 20 minutes. Even if your lunch break is only 30 minutes long, you can fit in a 20-minute stroll. For those of us who are able, walking is the foundation of cardiorespiratory fitness. With every step, you activate the pumps in your lower extremity and core muscles, power plants that expedite the return of blood to your heart.

3. If you are able, once or twice per week, challenge your cardiorespiratory system more intensively.

    a. Go for a long hike, preferably with hills. Walk at a much faster pace than in your daily walks. Every stride puts more spring in your step. If you swing your arms back and forth exuberantly, you will feel your whole body pulsate with the thrill of rhythmic exertion.

    b. Once your fitness level is fairly high—when a long fast walk becomes easy—try high intensity interval training (HIIT) for 20 minutes on a bike or an exercise cycle, on an elliptical trainer, or on a treadmill.

        (1) Do five minutes of warmup: going slowly at first, but at a gradually increasing pace each minute.

        (2) Beginning at the 5-minute point, do a 20 to 30 second burst (moving your legs as fast as possible) followed immediately by 90 to 100 seconds at a leisurely pace.

        (3) Repeat step (2) at the 7-, 9-, 11-, and 13-minute points, then

        (4) Do a 5-minute cooldown at a gradually declining pace.

4. If your strength training workout is well-organized, try to perform it with minimal rest time between sets. By moving from exercise to exercise as quickly as possible, you are doing another form of High Intensity Interval Training. Your heart rate will peak during the lifting phase of each exercise

and decline slightly during the short interval between each set of exercises. If you train in this manner, your heart rate and your rate of breathing will remain at elevated levels for the entire workout.

5. Monitor your heart rate periodically throughout the day. Many contemporary electronic devices track your heart rate and other fitness parameters continuously. By checking this data every few hours, you will soon discover how and when your heart rate changes throughout the day.

As your cardiorespiratory fitness improves, you will find the daily physical tasks of life become easier to complete, your energy levels stay higher, and you sleep more soundly. Although doing cardiorespiratory exercises is not the most important factor in decreasing your body fat, it is supremely important for the successful completion of many other physiological processes and meaningful activities in your life.

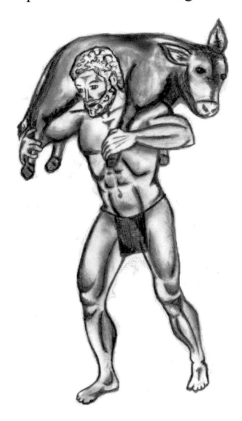

Milo of Croton

Five-Time Olympic Wrestling Champion

Chapter 9

Whole-Body, Strength-for-Life® Training

Some people who engage in strength training devote their attention primarily to the muscles of the arms, legs, chest, shoulders, and upper back. They treat "core" muscles and cardiorespiratory muscles as second-thought citizens, relegating them to the end of their workouts. As a result, often they perform exercises for these critical muscle groups hastily; or they forget them entirely. I hope, after reading the previous chapters of this book, you feel that challenging your core and cardiorespiratory muscles is just as important as training the larger and more glamorous muscles of your limbs.

Personally, I do the majority of core muscle training at the beginning my workouts. When I challenge these middle-of-the body muscles first, they feel loose, strong, and well-prepared for their crucial supportive functions in all subsequent exercises for the upper and lower limbs. In addition, as described in Chapter 8, I integrate cardiorespiratory conditioning throughout the performance of my strength training workouts. Thus, to best of my ability, I endeavor to practice whole-body strength training, that is, follow a training plan in which I challenge all the muscle groups important to the function and health of the human body. It is time now to consider core and cardiorespiratory muscle training within the context of your entire training plan. Abdominal Strength for Life® is part of a much bigger picture: Whole-Body, Strength-for-Life® Training.

What is Strength Training?

Strength training is not synonymous with lifting weights.

If strength training is not simply lifting weights, what is it?

Before we attempt to answer this question, let's take a step back and try to answer a more fundamental question:

What is Strength?

Although you may not often consider it in this way, strength is an important quality of your health. If you lack strength, or if you have strength and then lose it, the quality of your life is diminished significantly. Physically, you may lose your personal independence, even the ability to clothe and bathe yourself. Psychologically, if you lose your strength, you lose your self-confidence, the ability to confront the challenges of your day, and perhaps even the compassion to think of others who need your help. Therefore, I submit the following definition of strength for your consideration.

> *Strength in terms of health is your capacity to create the physical, mental, and spiritual forces needed to exceed the demands of everyday tasks, to excel in your chosen activities, to consider the needs of others, and to stimulate growth and repair in your body.*

You create physical strength by training your skeletal muscles to contract and relax as you perform powerful, coordinated, and skillful movements. You create mental and spiritual strength by facing obstacles in your life with calmness, confidence, and bravery. Training yourself to develop these varied dimensions of strength enables you to carry out the required and desired actions of your life with excellence and without experiencing premature structural breakdowns in your body. You feel strong and healthy. Your potential for long-term vitality is enhanced greatly, relative to what it would have been, if you had let your strength slip away. Within the context of strength as defined above, I offer the following definition of

Whole-Body, Strength-for-Life® Training.

> *Whole-body, Strength-for-Life® Training is an organized regimen of exercises in which you perform repeated muscular movements against various forms of resistance. The primary objectives of strength training exercises are to cause beneficial changes in bodily tissues, such as, increased bone and muscle mass, and changes in bodily functions, such as, increased strength and flexibility, improved circulation, deeper respirations, decreased*

*blood pressure, and enhanced agility and coordination. These
positive changes stimulate efficient function in all organ systems
of your body and enable you to perform your favorite physical
activities as well as possible for as long in life as possible.*

Three aspects of this definition of strength training are unique. First, the compound adjective "Whole-Body" emphasizes that this brand of training must always include stimulation for all muscle groups of your body, including the often-neglected muscles of your neck, hips, and cardiorespiratory system. Secondly, "for-Life" has two distinctly different implications: (1) that you should do this training for as long in your life as possible and (2) that doing these exercises will add liveliness to every day of your life. Third, when strength training exercises are executed with excellence, they improve the function in every other organ system of your body. Thus, in every repetition of every exercise, you are striving for whole-body health.

How Does Strength Training help you become Leaner for Life?

By executing the intense physical movements required in strength training, you expend more calories of energy than if you were sitting at a computer for the same period of time. However, as with cardiorespiratory conditioning, the number of additional calories you burn while doing a strength training workout is usually exceeded by the number of additional calories you will soon consume because that workout stimulated increasing hunger. You are reminded again, therefore, that you should not depend exclusively upon exercise to burn extra fat your body may be hoarding. But, unlike cardiorespiratory exercise, there are at least two ways in which strength training does help you become leaner: by increasing your muscle mass and by developing the strength in the core muscles that sustain excellent posture.

If you execute an organized strength training program consistently for a year, you may gain five to ten pounds of muscle mass. Even if your total body fat remains unchanged, your body fat percentage will decrease. And, if you study honest, 21st Century nutritional research and put its principles into your dietary practice, your body fat mass will decline as well. You should be able to verify you are leaner by having your body composition tested at your doctor's office.

If you perform all the core strengthening exercises described and illustrated in this book, one of the outstanding health benefits you will notice is that your posture is improved significantly. When you look in the mirror, your shoulders will appear more balanced. Your friends may say you look taller. You can verify that you are leaner by measuring the circumference of your waist at the level of the navel and comparing that result with the initial measurement taken before you began the Abdominal Strength for Life® program. Over the past thirty years in the Strength for Life® Health and Fitness Center, trainees average a waist circumference reduction of one inch after three months of consistent training.

Having defined "strength" and "strength training", I offer now the definitions and principles of training that I have developed and used for more than three decades while teaching in the Strength for Life® Health and Fitness Center.

Strength for Life® Training Definitions and Principles

A. **The Repetition**

1. **Definition #1: The primary functional unit of a strength training exercise is the repetition**. A repetition is not defined by the movement of a machine or a dumbbell; it is defined by the movements of your target muscles in each particular exercise.

2. **SfL Training Principle #1: Every repetition consists of two phases: a contraction phase and an extension phase.**

   a. The contraction phase begins with your target muscle(s) in a fully stretched position. Once you initiate movement, this phase continues until you have contracted your target muscle(s) to a fully shortened position.

      (1) The "fully stretched position" is the point at which you feel your target muscle(s) is (are) stretched to the maximal degree which is safe.

      (2) The "fully shortened position" is when you feel your target muscle(s) is (are) contracted as completely and as intensively as feels safe.

b. The extension phase is the return from contraction. After pausing in the fully contracted position, you move your target muscle(s) back slowly to a fully stretched position.

3. **SfL Training Principle #2: In every repetition, there should be a momentary pause in movement of the target muscle(s) at the end of each phase, that is, in the fully contracted position and again in the fully extended position.** A pause at the end of each phase facilitates the development of maximal strength and flexibility from every repetition you perform.

   a. The pause at the end of the contraction phase allows you an instant to concentrate and feel your target muscle(s) contract more intensely and more completely than if you were to bounce immediately into the extension phase. Creating an intense muscular contraction builds more muscle strength and size than rushing to do more repetitions in slipshod form.

   b. A pause at the end of the extension phase allows you a moment to feel the sensation of a complete stretch in the target muscle(s). This instant of motionless stretch increases flexibility in the tendons of your target muscle(s) before you begin the next repetition.

4. **SfL Training Principle #3: The optimal breathing pattern for all strength training exercises is as follows:**

   a. **In the fully stretched beginning position, inhale before initiating any movement.**

   b. **Begin to exhale as soon as you begin the contraction phase.**

   c. **Continue to exhale throughout the contraction phase until you reach the peak contraction position at the endpoint of that phase.** Therefore, the rate of contraction is synchronous with the rate of breathing; it takes as long to exhale completely as it does to contract your target muscle(s) completely.

   d. **Pause momentarily.**

e. **Begin to inhale slowly as you begin the extension phase by lengthening your target muscle(s) slowly.** It takes as long to complete the extension phase as it does to exhale completely.

f. **Pause momentarily in the fully stretched position again and savor the sensations in your target muscles before you initiate the contraction phase of the next repetition.**

g. The primary rationale for this breathing pattern is to prevent a Valsalva Maneuver in which blood flow to the heart is compromised and blood pressure increases dramatically for a few seconds. Competitive weight lifters may use the Valsalva Maneuver to create suddenly increased force to execute an extremely heavy lift. However, for those of us who do non-competitive strength training for lifetime health, avoiding Valsalva is a very wise choice. In addition, the rhythmic breathing pattern described above creates a steady pace for coordinated muscular movement throughout both phases of every repetition of every exercise.

h. Depending on your individual training goal for each specific exercise, continue to perform superb repetitions in the smooth, coordinated, and controlled manner described above until you complete…

B. **The Set.**

1. **Definition #2. For each specific strength training exercise, a set is a group of repetitions performed consecutively, with excellence, and throughout a full range of motion until you can no longer execute another full repetition**. When your target muscle(s) is (are) this fatigued, you have performed a strength training set. In completing this set, you have fulfilled the goal of challenging your target muscles to contract more intensively and lengthen more completely than they do in the ordinary activities of daily life. The process of challenging your muscles in this way is termed overloading. When you perform strength training exercises with this degree of intensity, and if your diet supplies the nutrients you need, you stimulate physiological factors that cause increases in your muscle and bone

mass, in the strength and flexibility of your muscles, tendons, and ligaments, and in your coordination and agility.

2. The number of repetitions in a set is highly dependent upon your goals and your strength and fitness level. If you are a beginning trainee, a typical set for you might be 10 to 20 repetitions with a relatively light weight. As an advanced trainee, you might use a moderately heavy weight with which you can complete only 4 to 6 repetitions. However, whether you do 4 repetitions in a set or 20, your goal is the same: challenge your target muscle(s) to contract a little more forcefully and stretch a little more completely than they are required to do in the physical activities of your everyday life. Demand this of your body consistently and it will respond by growing to be stronger and more flexible.

3. **SfL Training Principle #4: <u>Progressive</u> resistance training is the key to making ongoing improvements in your strength and fitness.** After the first few months of consistent strength training, you will be stronger, more flexible, and more agile. Your level of cardiorespiratory fitness will be higher. At this stage, however, your body will have adapted to the physical demands of your initial training program. You will not continue progressing toward your personal health goals, if you continue only to exercise in the same way you did as a beginning trainee. If you want to continue making health gains, you must increase the demands of your training somewhat. This is what is meant by the term progressive resistance training. What types of adjustments can you implement to make your training more progressive?

    a. Increase the number of repetitions you perform in each exercise. You should have been doing this all along.
    b. Increase the amount of resistance in each exercise. You should have been doing this all along, too.
    c. Increase the number of sets you perform of each exercise. If you are an intermediate or advanced level trainee, you will often perform more than one set of a particular exercise. The purpose of performing multiple sets of a specific exercise is to challenge the target muscles of that exercise more intensively than you can by doing only one set.

If you perform multiple sets strategically, you will create greater overload upon your target muscle(s), which will stimulate greater increases in muscle and bone growth. Strategies for organizing sets of strength training exercises are known as systems.

The three adjustments you can make in your training, as described in a, b, and c above, are all quantitative changes. You increase the physical demands of your training by increasing the amounts of weight you use, the quantity of repetitions you do, and/or the quantity of sets of repetitions you perform. But there is one other method to increase the intensity of your training which is qualitative, more important, and usually overlooked: your level of mental focus upon your target muscles as you perform each repetition of every exercise. This leads us to...

d. **SfL Training Principle #5: How intensively you focus your mind upon the sensations you feel in your target muscles as you perform a strength training exercise is the most important determinant of how the intensively you can contract and how fully you can extend those muscles.** What you are thinking about as you do strength training exercises has a profound effect upon your ability to stretch and strengthen the muscles upon which you depend to live your life with vigor. If you concentrate as you train, you will not only increase your muscle and bone mass, you will develop ever-greater control over the movements and functions of your body. How you perform an exercise and what you are thinking about as you perform that exercise, say volumes about you. Or, as we say at the Strength for Life® Health and Fitness Center:

Every millimeter of movement of every repetition of every exercise is an opportunity for personal artistic expression.

C. Systems

1. A system is the way in which the set or sets of specific exercises are grouped.

2. If you do only one set of each exercise, you are using a Single-Set System.

129

3. If you do two sets of an exercise, you are employing a Two-Set System with that specific exercise. Doing two or more sets of an exercise is another quantitative way to increase the demand of your strength training program.

4. If you do three sets of an exercise, you are using a Three-Set or Tri-Set System. Four sets, Quad-Set System, etc. In most cases, only advanced bodybuilders or competitive lifting athletes utilize more than three- or four-set systems.

5. Depending upon your fitness goals, you can arrange multiple sets of strength training exercises in a variety of systems.

    a. Serial System: perform two or more sets of the same exercise with a brief (1-3 minute) rest between sets. To make your training more progressive, increase the resistance for each set after the first. As you increase the resistance(s) for a second and/or third set, you will not be able to complete as many repetitions as you did in the first set.

    b. Superset System: perform a set of one exercise; move immediately to a different exercise and perform a set; move immediately back to the first exercise for a second set; move immediately back to the second exercise for a second set. As with the Serial System, you will probably increase the resistance and complete fewer repetitions with each successive set.

The superset system can be used by alternating between three or even four different exercises and with three, four, or even five sets of each exercise. This system has the added advantage of making your strength training workout a cardiorespiratory workout. If you move between the sets of exercises without resting, you will elevate your heart rate to a challenging training level. Your heart rate will remain at a high level until you complete the entire sequence of multiple sets of multiple exercises, which could take 25 or 30 minutes. Obviously, it will not be safe for you to attempt such intensive training until you have developed advanced levels of strength and cardiorespiratory fitness.

Even when you use multiple-set systems, it is important always to remind yourself that, during time you are performing an exercise, how well you concentrate on feeling your target muscles is paramount.

The next level of strength training organization is…

D. **The Workout**

1. **A Workout is your short-term training plan, the manner in which you arrange all the exercises which you intend to complete during one continuous period of time**. It can be as short as 20 minutes or as long as one or even two hours. The following two pages are examples of two separate workout plans for a beginning level trainee.

2. A workout is not a random grouping of exercises. It is a planned sequence of exercise challenges organized to stimulate growth in muscle and bone tissue, to enhance your cardiorespiratory capacity, to improve your flexibility, posture, coordination, and agility, and to enable you to perform the other physical tasks of your life with power and elegance. An example of a strategic workout plan could be as follows.

a. Warmup Exercises: 10 minutes of low-level, cardiorespiratory exercise to stimulate a mild increase in your heart rate and the depth of your respirations.

b. Core exercises: 10-15 minutes of exercises for the lower torso/hip complex to be certain these muscle groups are well-prepared for their supportive functions in the subsequent strength exercises.

c. Strength Exercises: 30-40 minutes of strength training exercises, moving from the largest muscles (such as the leg and hip muscles) at the beginning of this sequence to the smallest muscles (such as arms and neck) toward the end.

d. Stretching/Cooldown Exercises: 5-10 minutes of easy flexibility exercises to wind down from this workout and prepare for the next one.

Strength for Life® Training Plan & Log   Name_____ Workout # 1A   Year ____
Training Stage: 1 Beginning

Exercises		Date >		/		/		/		/	
Equipment Settings__/	Set #	Target Reps	Wt	Reps	Wt	Reps	Wt	Reps	Wt	Reps
I. Warmup											
Bike___/TM/Elliptical/ 5 min.											
Upper Body Ergometer/ 5 min. Seat___/Floor___/Arm___											
II. "Core" Exercises											
Lower Abdominal Curl	1	10								
Upper Abdominal Curl	1	10-20								
Diagonal Abdominal Curl	1R/1L	10-20								
Abdominal Vacuum	1	10								
Side Jackknife	1R/1L	10-20								
Pointer	R/L	10/10								
III. Strength Exercises											
Leg Press Sled___	1	10-20								
Calf Raise/ Shoulder Pad___	1	10-20								
Hip Extension/ Pad___ Center Pin____ Platform_____	1R/1L	10-15								
Lat Pulldown/ Knee Pad____ Grips_____	1	10-15								
Incline Press Seat_____ Grips___	1	10-15								
Rotary Torso Seat____ Rotation___ _°	1R/1L	10-15								
Back Extension Footplate___ Back Pad_____ Start____ End____	1	10-20								
Triceps Press Seat____	1	10-15								
Dumbbell Biceps Curl	1	10-15								
Neck Extension & Rotation / Prone on bench	1 / 1	10-15 / 10-15								
IV. Cardio/Agility											
V. Cooldown/Stretching											

| Exercises | | Date > | | / | | / | | / | | / | |
Equipment Settings__/	Set #	Target Reps	Wt	Reps	Wt	Reps	Wt	Reps	Wt	Reps
I. Warmup										
Bike___/TM/Elliptical/ 5 min.										
Upper Body Ergometer/ 5 min. Seat / Floor / Arm___										
II. "Core" Exercises										
Lower Abdominal Curl	1	10								
Upper Abdominal Curl	1	10-20								
Diagonal Abdominal Curl	1R/1L	10-20								
Abdominal Vacuum	1	10								
Side Jackknife	1R/1L	10-20								
Pointer	R/L	10/10								
III. Strength Exercises										
Leg Extension Back Pad___/ Shin Pad___	1	10-20								
Leg Curl Ankle Pad __	1	10-20								
Hip Flexion Pad___ Center Pin__ Platform___	1R/1L	10-15								
Rowing Seat__ Chest Pad ___ Grips____	1	10-15								
Chest Press Seat___ Grips____	1	10-15								
Pullover Seat___	1R/1L	10-15								
Chest Fly Seat___ (Keep Footbar Down)	1	10-15								
Triceps Extension Seat___ / Back Pad___	1	10-15								
Dumbbell Hammer Curls	1	10-15								
Neck Lateral Flexion & Rotation / Sidelying on bench	1R/1L 1R/1L	10-15 10-15								
IV. Cardio/Agility										
V. Cooldown/ Stretching										

133

E. **Weekly, Monthly, Yearly, and Lifetime Strength Training Plans**

1. Your weekly training plan consists of the days each week in which you plan to perform your workouts.

    a. A general guideline is that one strength training workout each week is enough to keep your body from decaying too quickly, but not frequent enough to improve your fitness and strength significantly. However, if you have a very physically demanding job, one workout weekly might be enough to help you feel somewhat more flexible.

    b. Two workouts per week should be considered as the minimum frequency for making good progress toward your strength and fitness goals. Ideally, you would have two separate workouts that you could perform on an alternating basis, such as depicted in the training plans on the previous two pages. In this way, you would not be doing exactly the same exercises on every workout day.

    c. Three strength training workouts per week is an excellent weekly plan for people who are busy with their careers, family needs, and other responsibilities. Ideally, you would space your training sessions apart, resulting in a day or two between each workout. In the beginning months, you could continue alternating two separate workouts. However, at some point you should become more adventuresome and add a third distinct workout. This will add not only more variety to your training, but also allow you to develop more dimensions of health and fitness.

    d. As you advance further in your pursuit of strength and fitness, you might consider adding a fourth workout to your weekly plan, if your schedule permits. This need not be a formal strength training workout but, instead, some other form of physical exertion. A brisk walk or run, a bike ride, and working up a sweat in your yard or garden are good examples.

2. During some months of the year, you monthly training plan might only be a collection of four or five weekly plans. However, the events of your monthly calendar might include a vacation or a business trip. In cases such as

this, use an out-of-the-ordinary event as an opportunity to try vigorous activities which you have never attempted before or which you have not done for a long time. You might be surprised at how strong and agile your newly strengthened body feels when you challenge yourself with a physical pursuit to which you are not accustomed.

3. Your yearly strength training plan can include a great deal of variation from month to month or season to season. If you ride your bike with gusto all summer, you might decrease your lower extremity exercises in the gym during that period. If you vacation in the South during the winter months, you should search for alternative places and ways to keep your body moving during that season. You may even consider a month with no formal strength training while you attend a yoga retreat. Creating variety in your yearly fitness plan is termed periodization.

4. Your lifetime training plan is very simple; you are going to exert yourself as physically, as intelligently, as vigorously, and as consistently as you possibly can for as long in your life as you are able. If you engage in lifetime strength training, at whatever level you are capable, you will be amazed at how well you are able to perform physical activities which your less-active contemporaries abandoned decades ago. And do not be surprised if you feel the urge to take up other physical challenges you never imagined you would undertake previously. You and your life are lively. You are reaping the reward of fabulous health because you have cultivated your Strength for Life.

Throughout human history, the relative scarcity of food and the physical demands of daily labor kept the majority of us lean. Today, however, in a sedentary society littered with industrial foodstuffs that raise our blood sugar levels, inflame our GI tracts, and cause our bodies to store excessive amounts of fat, attaining and maintaining a healthful body composition is a real challenge.

If we cave in to the twin temptations of eating fat-gaining foodstuffs and exerting ourselves physically as little as possible, we will be able to "get by"—for a while. The massive economies of contemporary civilization want us to stay alive, so we continue to buy their stuff, whether we need it or not. Their conveniences, their toxic foodstuffs, and their drugs can keep us alive—at least long enough to buy our share of what they want to sell us. By following their prescriptions for "the Good Life" during the past 75 years, too many of us have become the helpless, passive victims of obesity and physical weakness. Those of us who remain passive, who allow these trends to continue, will remain as hopeless colonists who have sacrificed all hope for the joy and freedom of vibrant health.

You, by contrast—in the revolutionary act of reading this book—have decided to fight for your personal vitality.

It has been and remains the major purpose of this book to provide inspiration to you and to every reader who seeks the freedom of good health by developing leaner and stronger core muscles within the context whole-body exercise and an active lifestyle. Achieving this goal is not easy for any of us. However, we must remind ourselves that our objectives are not to be perfectly lean and pre-eminently strong. Rather, the essential goals for each one us are to be <u>leaner</u> and to be <u>stronger</u>. These are goals which every one of us can strive to attain.

May you discover and savor the joy of striving for leaner and stronger abdominals within the context of becoming a leaner, stronger, and more thoughtful person.

If I have learned three things during my career as a healthcare professional, they are:

1. To continue growing as a person, I must continue striving to learn;

2. I have made many mistakes and I continue to make many mistakes;

3. When I listen, I learn a great deal from virtually every person I encounter.

If you have comments, suggestions, criticisms, or corrections regarding anything you have read in this book, I am eager to learn from you. Please contact me at:

Drjosef@StrengthForLife.com.

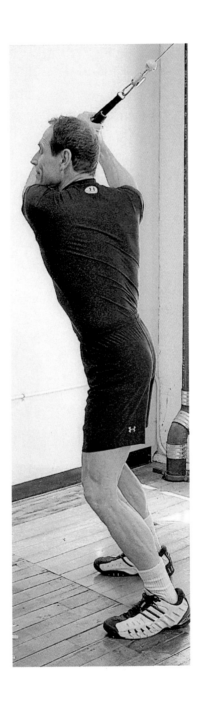

About the Author

Even in his early childhood, Josef Arnould enjoyed the quest for physical fitness. Whether it was catching snakes, climbing trees, throwing rocks and snowballs, or hitting baseballs, he loved the thrill of physical exertion. As a voracious teenage reader, he was stimulated especially by the relationship of good nutrition to successful athletic performance.

After graduating from Princeton University and Framingham State University, with bachelor's and master's degrees in English and Language Arts respectively, he entered Palmer College of Chiropractic with a career ambition of helping others achieve good health. In the curriculum at Palmer, he studied anatomy, physiology and nutrition in great depth.

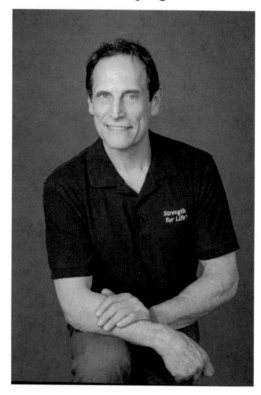

Upon receiving his doctorate in 1983, Dr. Arnould opened a clinic in Western Massachusetts. From his first days of practice, he was determined to fuse three natural disciplines of health: whole-body exercise; nutritious eating; and comprehensive chiropractic healthcare. To symbolize his commitment to this concept, he named his practice Strength for Life® Health and Fitness Center. Now in its 35th year, this clinic thrives as a community where people of all ages come to learn about exercising and eating intelligently and about receiving chiropractic care when necessary.

To share the knowledge and experience he had gained from many years of reading and teaching, as well as his lifelong love of exercise, Dr. Arnould composed a comprehensive textbook, *Stronger After 40: Strength Training as Healthcare for Women and Men in the 21st Century.* Published by Alward Publications in 2005, this work contains hundreds of photos and detailed explanations demonstrating how we can perform strength training and flexibility exercises safely and well, even if we are 80 or 90 years of age.

Now in his 70s, Dr. Arnould keeps us up-to-date in the exploding field of nutrition with an exciting new book, *American Diet Revolution!* which will be released in print by Morgan James Publishing on February 12, 2019. Much more than a manual of dietary advice, in this work we learn why and how, if we value our own health and the health of everyone we know and love, we must become activists about the foods we purchase and eat. Instead of an appeal for your relaxed consideration, this book inspires you to take action! To read a brief summary of *ADR!* or to pre-order a copy, go to StrengthForLife.com or to Amazon.com.

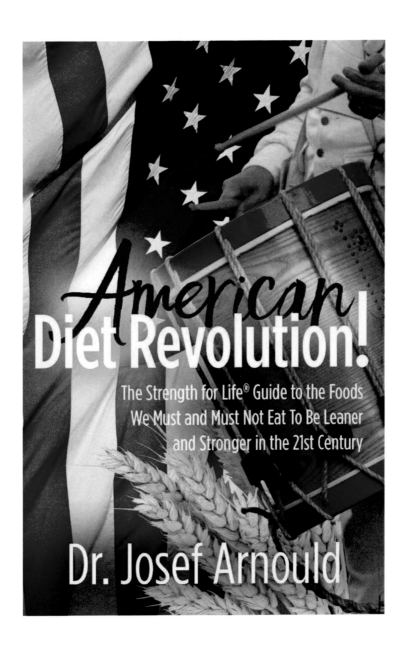

Made in the USA
Monee, IL
03 February 2020

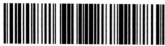